Principles of Renal Physiology

CHRISTOPHER J. LOTE

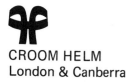

CROOM HELM
London & Canberra

© 1982 Christopher J. Lote
Croom Helm Ltd, Provident House, Burrell Row,
Beckenham, Kent BR3 1AT
Croom Helm Australia, PO Box 391,
Manuka, ACT 2603, Australia
Reprinted 1983

British Library Cataloguing in Publication Data

Lote, Christopher J.
   Principles of renal physiology.
   1. Kidneys
   I. Title
   612'.463   QP249

   ISBN 0-7099-0079-1

Printed and bound in Great Britain by
Biddles Ltd, Guildford and King's Lynn

CONTENTS

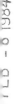
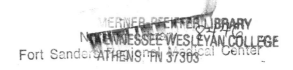

PREFACE

This book is based on the lecture course in renal physiology which I give to medical students at The University of Birmingham. The purpose of the book is primarily to set out the principles of renal physiology for preclinical medical students, and it is therefore concerned mainly with normal renal function. However, diseases or abnormalities in other body systems may lead to adaptations or modifications of renal function, so that a good knowledge of renal physiology is essential to the understanding of many disease states, for example, the oedema of heart failure or liver disease, or the consequences of haemorrhage and shock. The relationship of renal function to such conditions is included in the book, so that clinical students and medical practitioners should find it useful.

In order to avoid breaking up the text, I have not included references to every statement. Instead, there is a reading list at the end of each chapter, which in general includes review articles and recent papers to provide access to the current literature. Although the book is, as far as possible, a statement of known facts, it is not intended to be an over-simplification, and where there are areas of uncertainty these are pointed out.

The book could not have been written without the help and advice of friends and colleagues, and I particularly wish to thank Dr J. Coote of the Department of Physiology at Birmingham, and Professor R. Green of Manchester University Physiology Department, for reading and criticising the manuscript, and Dr M. Kendall of the Department of Therapeutics, University of Birmingham, for his help with Chapters 13 and 14.

Finally, my thanks to Miss Linda Hancocks for faultlessly typing the manuscript, and to the publishers for their patience.

TERMINOLOGY AND ABBREVIATIONS

General

ADH	Antidiuretic hormone (vasopressin)
ECG	Electrocardiogram
ERPF	Effective renal plasma flow
GFR	Glomerular filtration rate
RBF	Renal blood flow
RPF	Renal plasma flow

Units of Measurement

mosm	milliosmoles
mm Hg	millimetres of mercury (pressure measurement)
mM	millimoles/litre
mmol	millimoles
nm	nanometres (10^{-9} metres)
μm	micrometres (10^{-6} metres)

Symbols

Square brackets, thus [ ] denote concentration, e.g. plasma $[Na^+]$ = 140 mM means plasma sodium concentration = 140 mM.

1 THE BODY FLUIDS

Introduction

The body fluids can be considered to be distributed between two compartments, intracellular and extracellular. The extracellular compartment can in turn be divided into a number of sub-compartments. These are: (a) the plasma (extracellular fluid within the vascular system); (b) the interstitial fluid (extracellular fluid outside the vascular system, and functionally separated from it by the capillary endothelium); and (c) transcellular fluids. Transcellular fluid can be defined as extracellular fluid which is separated from the plasma by an additional epithelial layer, as well as by the capillary endothelium. Transcellular fluids have specialised functions, and include the fluid within the digestive and urinary tracts, the synovial fluid in the joints, the aqueous and vitreous humours in the eye, and the cerebrospinal fluid.

The environment in which our cells exist is not the environment of the outside of the body. The immediate environment of the cells is the extracellular fluid. This *internal environment* (a term first used by the nineteenth century French physiologist, Claude Bernard) provides the stable medium necessary for the normal functioning of the cells of the body. The internal environment maintains the correct concentrations of oxygen, carbon dioxide, ions and nutritional materials, for the normal functioning of the cells.

Maintenance of the constancy of the internal environment (which the American physiologist, Walter B. Cannon, called 'homeostasis') is ensured by several body systems. For example, the partial pressures of oxygen and carbon dioxide are regulated by the lungs. The kidneys play a vital role in homeostasis. In fact, they can reasonably be regarded as the most important regulatory organs for controlling the internal environment, since they control not only the concentration of waste products of metabolism, but also the osmolality, volume, acid-base status and ionic composition of the extracellular fluid, and indirectly the kidneys regulate these same variables within the cells.

Much of this book is devoted to an examination of the ways in which the kidneys perform these regulatory functions. First, however, it is necessary to examine the normal composition of the body fluids.

Body Water

Water is the major component of the human body, and in any individual body water content stays remarkably constant from day to day. However, there is considerable variability in the water content of different individuals, and this variability is due to differences in the amount of adipose tissue (fat) in different people.

In a 70 kg man of average build, the body water will constitute 63 per cent of the body weight, and thus there will be 45 ℓ of total body water (TBW). In a woman of the same weight, only about 52 per cent (36 ℓ) of the body weight will be water. This difference is due to the fact that women have more adipose tissue than men, and the water content of adipose tissue is very low (about 10 per cent).

In obese people, fat is a major constituent of the body (second only to water), and even 'slim' people have considerable quantities of fat. We can regard the fat as non-functional (storage) tissue. The functional tissue of the body can be regarded as fat-free: the percentage of water in the fat-free tissue is extremely constant, both within an individual from day to day, and between individuals. The percentage water in this 'lean body mass' is 73 per cent.

Body Fluid Osmolality

The exchange of water between the different body fluid compartments is facilitated by two forces: hydrostatic pressure and osmotic pressure. In order to understand osmotic pressure, consider a container of water, separated into two compartments by a membrane permeable to water. The water molecules will be moving at random (Brownian motion), and some of them will be moving across the membrane by diffusion; the rate of diffusion in each direction will be equal, so that net flux is zero. Now suppose that a solute is added to one compartment. The addition of solutes to water reduces the random movement (activity) of the water molecules, and consequently the diffusion of water from the side containing the solute to the side containing only water will be reduced. There will then be a net flux of water from the pure water side to the solution side of the membrane (Figure 1.1). We can measure this osmotic effect as an *osmotic pressure*, by determining the hydrostatic pressure which must be applied to the compartment containing solute, to prevent the net entry of water. This hydrostatic pressure is equal to the *osmotic pressure* of the solution.

Figure 1.1: A container divided into two compartments by a membrane permeable to water, but impermeable to some solutes. (Such membranes are termed 'semi-permeable'.) (a) When there is only water in the container, the unidirectional water fluxes (represented by the arrows) are equal, so that the net flux of water is zero. (b) If a solute to which the membrane is impermeable is added to one compartment of the container, the activity of the water molecules on the side containing the solute is reduced, so that the unidirectional water flux from that side is reduced. The unidirectional water flux into the solute-containing side continues as before, so that there is a net flux into the solute-containing side, which creates a hydrostatic pressure difference (h). This hydrostatic pressure is equal to the *osmotic pressure* of the solution. Alternatively, the osmotic pressure of the solution could be measured by determining the hydrostatic pressure which must be applied to the solute-containing side to prevent the net influx of water to this compartment. Water moves from an area of *low* osmolality to one of *higher* osmolality.

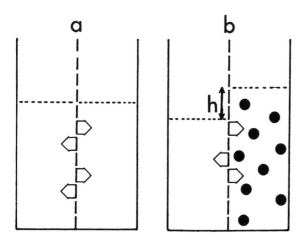

Units of Osmotic Measurement

From the foregoing, it is apparent that, like hydrostatic pressure, osmotic pressure could be expressed as mm Hg. A more useful unit, however, is the osmole, and in physiology osmolality is usually expressed as milliosmoles/kg H_2O. The osmole is analogous to the mole (and, for non-dissociable substances, is *identical* to the mole, i.e. it is 1 gram molecular weight of a non-dissociable molecule). For molecules which dissociate, each particle derived from the molecule contributes to the osmotic pressure, and so to calculate the osmolality from the molality, it is necessary to multiply by the number of particles. Suppose a molecule dissociates into n ions; then osmolality is given by osmolality (mosmoles/kg H_2O) = $n \times$ molar

concentration (mmole/kg H_2O)

It should be noted that the units of osmolality (and molality) refer to the concentration per unit weight of *solvent* (water). This is in contrast to osmolarity (and molarity) which refers to the (os)molar concentration per litre of solution (i.e. water + solute), so units of osmolarity are mosmol/ℓ. Osmolality is the preferred measurement, although in practice the difference between the two terms when dealing with physiological solute concentrations is very small.

Isotonicity and Isosmoticity

If red blood cells are suspended in distilled water, water enters the cells by osmosis and the cells swell and burst. This is haemolysis. If the cells are suspended in a solution which does not cause any change in the cell volume, such a solution is termed *isotonic*. The most widely used isotonic solution is 0.9 per cent saline. Five per cent dextrose is also isotonic. Both of these solutions have an osmolality of about 285 mosmol/kg H_2O, as do the cell contents and the plasma. Solutions having the same osmolality are termed *isosmotic*. However, although different isotonic solutions are isosmotic, solutions which are isosmotic to the plasma are not necessarily isotonic. This can be demonstrated if red cells are suspended in an isosmotic urea solution. The cells swell and haemolyse, just as they do in distilled water. This occurs because urea can readily cross cell membranes and thus equilibrates across the membrane to reach the same concentration on each side, so that the osmotic effect of the urea is cancelled and the osmolality of the other intracellular solutes causes the cell to swell (Figure 1.2).

Whether a solute is an 'ineffective' osmole in this way depends not only on the solute, but also on the properties of the membrane. Thus urea is an 'ineffective osmole' across the cell membrane, because it diffuses so rapidly, whereas Na^+ is an effective osmole. In contrast, the capillary membrane is much more permeable than the cell membrane, so *all* the solutes in the plasma except the plasma proteins are 'ineffective osmoles' in relation to the capillary walls. An 'effective osmole' is a solute which when placed on one side of a semi-permeable membrane, will tend to cause water movement across that membrane. An 'ineffective osmole' is one which, when placed on one side of a semi-permeable membrane, will itself rapidly diffuse across the membrane.

Figure 1.2: A container divided into two compartments by a semi-permeable membrane, as in Figure 1.1. (a) Net flux of water is zero, as in Figure 1.1a. (b) Addition to the compartment on the right of a solute which can readily cross the membrane, does not significantly alter the net water flux, because the solute rapidly equilibrates across the membrane (i.e. reaches the same concentration on each side). A solute which behaves in this way is termed an 'ineffective osmole'.

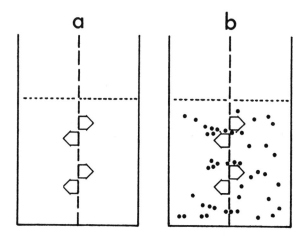

Normal Body Fluid Osmolality

The body fluid osmolality is maintained remarkably constant, at 280-290 mosmol/kg H_2O. How this constancy is achieved is the subject of a later chapter of this book. However, at this stage it should be noted that, in general, intracellular and extra-cellular fluid osmolalities are identical, because water can readily cross the cell membranes.

The Distribution of Ions across Biological Membranes

Because of their random thermal motion (Brownian movement), the individual molecules of dissolved substances are continually diffusing, so that there are no concentration differences between different parts of a solution. (If the concentration of a dissolved substance is higher in one region than another, then molecules will diffuse in both directions, but more will diffuse from the region of high concentration to the region of lower concentration than vice versa, so that the concentrations become equal.)

Biological membranes (e.g. cell membranes, capillary membranes) permit the diffusion of small molecules and ions through them. However, substances diffuse through biological membranes (particularly cell membranes) much more slowly than they diffuse freely in water, and different molecules and ions diffuse through membranes at different rates depending on their molecular weight, shape and charge. So the cell membrane is *selective*, allowing some molecules to pass much more readily than others. Some large molecules (e.g. proteins) diffuse across the cell membrane so slowly that the membrane is effectively impermeable to them.

The presence of such non-permeant ions (e.g. proteins, which are generally anions at physiological pH) on one side of a membrane which is permeable to other ions, causes the unequal distribution of the diffusible ions — this is the *Gibbs-Donnan effect*. Ion distribution will be such that the products of the concentrations of diffusible ions on the two sides will be equal, i.e. if we call the two sides a and b

$$\begin{array}{ccc} \text{diffusible} & & \text{diffusible} \\ \text{cations}_{\text{(side a)}} & \times & \text{anions}_{\text{(side a)}} \end{array} = \begin{array}{ccc} \text{diffusible} & & \text{diffusible} \\ \text{cations}_{\text{(side b)}} & \times & \text{anions}_{\text{(side b)}} \end{array}$$

A consequence of this distribution is that the total number of ions on the side containing non-diffusible ions will be slightly greater than the total number of ions on the side containing only diffusible ions; so the osmotic pressure will be slightly greater on the side containing the non-diffusible ions.

Thus there is a slight imbalance of ions between the inside and outside of *capillaries*, due to the presence of non-diffusible plasma proteins within the capillaries (see p. 19).

Across *cell membranes*, however, the situation is more complicated. Cell membranes are permeable to K^+ and Cl^-, but much less permeable to Na^+ (Na^+ permeance is less than 1/50 that of K^+). In addition, there are *active* transport processes in the cell membrane, which actively extrude sodium and keep the intracellular sodium concentration very low. The active Na^+ pump also pumps K^+ into the cell, and since the pump uses ATP, it is a Na^+-K^+ ATPase. However, the permeability of the membrane to K^+ is so high that the pump has little effect on the K^+ distribution, whereas it has a very marked effect on Na^+ distribution.

Inside cells, there are proteins which have a net negative charge (protein anions). These will tend to cause the accumulation of positive ions inside the cell. Since Na^+ is actively kept out of the cell, K^+ enters. This makes the K^+ concentration inside very high and there will be some diffusion out down the concentration gradient, so that electrical neutrality will not be achieved and at equilibrium the cell will have a net negative charge (about -70 mV). Chloride will distribute passively across the cell membrane and so, because of the net negative charge inside the cell, there will be more chloride outside. Sodium is present in high concentration outside the cell because of the active sodium pump.

We might expect, as a result of the Gibbs-Donnan effect detailed above, that there would be more ions inside the cell than outside, because of the non-diffusible intracellular proteins. However these are balanced by sodium outside, which, because of the sodium pump, is effectively non-diffusible. If the sodium pump is chemically inhibited, sodium is no longer effectively non-diffusible, and so the cells swell by osmosis. Thus the Na^+ pump is essential for the osmotic stability of cells.

Fluid Exchanges between Body Compartments

Although the body fluid compartments have a relatively constant composition and are in equilibrium with each other, this equilibrium is not static, but dynamic. There is a continual internal fluid exchange, between the plasma and the interstitial fluid, and between the interstitial fluid and the cells.

Exchanges between Interstitial Fluid and Intracellular Fluid

Cell membranes have a much lower permeability than capillary endothelia to ions and water-soluble molecules. Nevertheless, water can freely cross cell membranes, so that intracellular and extracellular fluids are in osmotic equilibrium. Changes in the ionic content of the intracellular or extracellular fluid will lead to corresponding movements of water between the two compartments. Na^+ ions are the most important extracellular osmotically active ions, whereas K^+ ions are most important intracellularly. If we added more sodium to the extracellular fluid — e.g. by ingesting NaCl — the extra solute would osmotically attract water from the intracellular fluid until the osmolality of intra- and extracellular fluids was again equal, and the osmolalities of both compartments would be increased, even though the added solute was confined to the extracellular fluid.

Exchanges between the Plasma and Interstitial Fluid

The functionally important part of the vascular system, for this exchange to occur, is the capillaries. Water and electrolytes move

Figure 1.3: Fluid exchange between the plasma and interstitial fluid across the capillary wall. At the arteriolar end (on the left) the capillary hydrostatic pressure (P, 32 mm Hg) exceeds the osmotic pressure due to the plasma proteins (π, 25 mm Hg), so there is a loss of fluid from the capillary. At the venous end (on the right) the plasma protein osmotic pressure (π, 25 mm Hg) is greater than the hydrostatic pressure (P, 12 mm Hg), because hydrostatic pressure decreases along the capillary. Thus at the venous end, fluid re-enters the capillary.

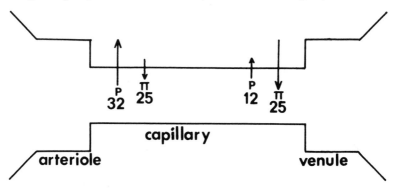

continuously through the capillary walls between the plasma and the interstitial fluid, in both directions. Most of this movement (90 per cent) occurs as a result of simple diffusion. In addition, there is a 10 per cent contribution to the movement by filtration – at the arteriolar end of a capillary, there is a gradient (of hydrostatic pressure) causing fluid filtration through the capillary wall from the vascular system into the interstitial fluid. At the venous end of the capillary, the filtration gradient (due to osmotic pressure) is directed *into* the capillary. This is illustrated in Figure 1.3. (In fact real capillaries, unlike the idealised capillary shown in the diagram, are perfused intermittently: at times when blood is flowing through the capillary, the hydrostatic pressure inside is high enough to cause transudation out of the capillary along its entire length. When flow stops, reabsorption occurs along the whole length of capillary. The overall effect is as if the capillaries behaved like the idealised capillary in Figure 1.3.)

The movement of fluid across the capillary endothelium in each direction has been estimated to be about 120 ℓ/min. Since the plasma volume is only 3 ℓ, it follows that the plasma water completely exchanges with the interstitial fluid every 1.5 seconds!

The diffusive flow is mainly dependent on the physical characteristics of the capillary endothelium, and the size and chemical nature of the solutes. Oxygen and carbon dioxide are lipid soluble and can therefore diffuse freely across the entire surface of the capillaries (since the cell membranes of the capillary endothelial cells, like all cell membranes, are composed mainly of lipid). Water, small molecules and ions pass through space (pores) between the capillary endothelial cells. Of the plasma constituents, only the plasma proteins are unable to cross the capillary walls, so the plasma proteins exert the osmotic effect across the capillary walls (i.e. are effective osmoles), which is responsible for the re-entry of fluid at the venous end of the capillaries to balance the fluid filtered out by the hydrostatic pressure gradient at the arterial end.

Let us examine the forces governing movements across the capillary wall in more detail.

The *hydrostatic pressure* within the capillary is about 32 mm Hg at the arterial end, and has fallen to about 12 mm Hg by the venous end. This pressure depends on:

(1) the arterial blood pressure;
(2) the extent to which the arterial pressure is transmitted to the capillaries – i.e. the arteriolar resistance;
(3) the venous pressure.

Normally, the pressure at the arterial end of the capillaries is closely regulated and stays virtually constant. However, alterations in venous pressure will produce changes in capillary hydrostatic pressure.

The *oncotic pressure* (plasma protein osmotic pressure) in the capillary is commonly stated to be 25 mm Hg. In fact the plasma proteins are responsible for there being an osmotic pressure difference of 25 mm Hg between the capillaries and the interstitial fluid, but it is not strictly true to say that the pressure is entirely due to plasma proteins. The plasma proteins exert an osmotic effect of about 17 mm Hg. However, they have a net negative charge, and since the capillary endothelium is a semipermeable membrane, the plasma proteins cause an imbalance of diffusible ions across the capillary wall, so that there are more ions (mainly sodium) inside the capillary than outside. This imbalance is responsible for a further 8 mm Hg osmotic pressure, making a total osmotic pressure of 25 mm Hg.

In the interstitial fluid, there are usually small amounts of plasma proteins which have escaped from the capillary. These make little contribution to the balance of forces across the capillary endothelium, but this situation may change if the permeability of the capillaries to proteins increases for any reason, or if the removal of proteins from the interstitial fluid by the lymphatic system is reduced (see below).

It is very difficult to measure the interstitial fluid hydrostatic pressure (sometimes called the tissue turgor pressure). Estimates vary from a figure of 4 mm Hg, to about -8 mm Hg; it seems reasonable to regard the tissue hydrostatic pressure as approximately zero.

Lymphatic System

The lymphatic system is a network of thin vessels (resembling veins) which begins as lymphatic capillaries in almost all the organs and tissues of the body, and which eventually drains into the venous system in the neck. Although the lymph capillaries are blind-ended, they have walls which are very permeable, so that all the interstitial fluid components are able to enter them. The lymphatics thus provide a mechanism for returning to the vascular system those plasma proteins which have escaped from blood capillaries.

Blockage of the lymph drainage (e.g. as a result of carcinoma or other disease) causes the local accumulation of fluid (oedema); this is primarily because of the accumulation of proteins in the interstitial spaces, so that the oncotic pressure difference between blood capillaries and interstitial fluid is reduced, and consequently the reabsorption of tissue fluid into the blood capillaries is impaired.

Fluid Exchanges between the Body and the External Environment

The body fluid is continually exchanging with the external environment, but the constancy of body weight from day to day indicates that there is equality of fluid intake and output.

Water intake: the following are typical figures for water intake per 24 hrs.

drinking	1500 mℓ
food	500 mℓ
metabolism	400 mℓ
Total	2400 mℓ

The metabolically-derived water comes from the oxidation of food substances, e.g. the reaction for glucose oxidation is:

$$C_6H_{12}O_6 + 6O_2 \rightarrow 6CO_2 + 6H_2O$$

Water output: this occurs from the body by several routes: the typical figures per 24 hrs are

lungs	400 mℓ
skin	400 mℓ
faeces	100 mℓ
urine	1500 mℓ
Total	2400 mℓ

The loss from the lungs occurs because air, as it enters the lungs during inspiration, becomes saturated with water vapour as it passes along the respiratory tract. Some of this water is then lost during expiration. The figure of 400 mℓ is really the minimum loss. In hot dry environments, or in sub-zero temperatures (when the air is very dry because the water vapour has condensed and frozen), the loss of water from the lungs can be considerably greater than 400 mℓ.

The water loss through the skin (400 mℓ) is termed 'insensible perspiration', and occurs at an almost constant rate. It is not sweat. Sweating, or 'sensible perspiration', represents an additional loss, of up to 5 ℓ per hour (in order to dissipate excess heat and so maintain constancy of body temperature). The faecal water loss (100 mℓ) can be greatly increased in diarrhoea, which can lead to the loss of several litres per day.

All of the losses mentioned so far (lungs, skin, faeces) can be regarded as *disturbances* of the body fluid volume. In contrast, the urinary loss, which is normally about 1,500 mℓ/24 hrs, can be as little as 300 mℓ, or as much as about 23 litres. It is *adjusted according to the needs of the body* – i.e. the renal fluid output is regulatory (see Chapter 7). However, water intake can be reduced to zero (so that the only water input is that derived from metabolism), whereas the losses from lungs, skin, faeces and kidneys can never be less than about 1200 mℓ/day. This means that survival without any dietary water is only possible for a short time (generally less than one week).

Ionic Composition of the Body Fluids

Because the body fluid osmolality is regulated and normally kept

Figure 1.4: Ionic concentrations of the body fluids (mmol/ℓ), and the exchanges between body fluid compartments. The figures for plasma are given, in parentheses, as concentration per litre of plasma water. These values are higher than the concentrations in total plasma, because the ions are present only in the aqueous phase, but 70 mℓ/ℓ of plasma is protein and lipid. Thus the 930 mℓ of water per litre of plasma contains sodium at a concentration of 153 mmol/ℓ H_2O so the concentration of sodium in total plasma is 153 × 930/1000 mmol/ℓ plasma = 142 mmol/ℓ. The compartment volumes indicated are typical values for a 70 kg man. Intracellular fluids in different tissues differ slightly in composition. The values given are for skeletal muscle cells. Note that Na^+ and K^+ are actively transported across the cell membrane (although potassium also diffuses readily across this membrane). The protein constituents of the plasma and of intracellular fluid do not diffuse in significant amounts into the interstitial fluid.

| | PLASMA | INTERSTITIAL FLUID | INTRACELLULAR FLUID | TRANSCELLULAR FLUID | | |
				CSF	Gastric Juice	Ileac Secretion
Na^+	142.0 (153)	145.0	12.0	141.0	60.0	129.0
K^+	4.0 (4.3)	4.1	150.0	3.0	9.0	11.0
Cl^-	103.0 (109)	113.0	4.0	127.0	84.0	116.0
HCO_3^-	25.0 (26)	27.0	12.0	23.0	0.0	29.0
Proteins g/l	60.0	0.0	25.0	0.2	v. low	v. low
Osmolality mosmol/kg	280.0	280.0	280.0	280.0	280.0	280.0
Compartment Volume (1)	3.0	12.0	30.0	total transcellular fluid volume is estimated to be about 5% of total body water or 2.251		

(note between intracellular and transcellular columns: "exchange regulated by specific transport processes")

constant, it is obvious that the body water content will depend on the overall ionic content of the body and the distribution of water between the body fluid compartments will depend on the distribution of ions (Figure 1.4). Quantitatively, the most important ions in the body fluids are sodium (the major extracellular ion) and potassium (the major intracellular ion).

Extracellular Fluid (ECF)

The major ions of the ECF are shown in Figure 1.4. Sodium (Na^+) is the most important cation; chloride (Cl^-) and bicarbonate (HCO_3^-) are the most important anions. The plasma proteins are also anions. In fact the colloids of plasma (i.e. the plasma proteins and lipids) occupy a significant volume (70 mℓ/litre), so that only 930 mℓ of each litre of plasma is water, and this can lead to errors in the measurement of other solute concentrations, particularly in pathological conditions involing hyperlipidaemia. Figure 1.4 shows the differences in solute concentrations in total plasma and in the plasma water, and it can be seen that the discrepancy is considerable.

Intracellular Fluid

Intracellular fluid composition is shown in Figure 1.4, but it should be noted that it is not the same throughout the body. Different types of cells have different compositions. Furthermore, each cell is compartmentalised and the different cellular sub-compartments have different compositions. Nevertheless, in all cells the most important cation, quantitatively, is K^+, and the most important anions are the intracellular proteins and phosphate.

Ion Exchanges between the Body and the External Environment

We saw on p. 17 that the *osmolality* of the extracellular fluid depends on the sodium content. Since body fluid osmolality is regulated (see Chapter 7) it follows that the extracellular fluid *volume* also depends on the sodium content of the organism (see also Chapter 8). In a 70 kg man of average build, there are about 4,000 mmoles of sodium, 2,500 mmoles of chloride and 400 mmoles of bicarbonate.

Potassium is the major ion of the intracellular fluid, and so the osmolality and volume of this body fluid compartment depend primarily on the potassium content. Our 70 kg average man contains about 4,000 mmoles of potassium, of which only about 50 mmoles are in the extracellular fluid (and therefore directly accessible to the kidneys).

The diet may contain widely varying amounts of both Na^+ and K^+. The average Western diet contains about 10 g NaCl per day (170 mmoles sodium), but a vegetarian diet may contain very little Na^+ and large quantities of K^+. Nevertheless in spite of this potentially enormous variation in dietary intake, the sodium and potassium contents of the body are normally kept constant. This regulation is brought about mainly by renal control of the tubular reabsorption of the filtered sodium. Much of the rest of this book is concerned directly or indirectly with this process. For potassium, the control is brought about by the tubular reabsorption of about 95 per cent of the filtered K^+ and then the secretion of a variable amount of K^+.

The ability of the body to regulate the plasma K^+ concentration depends to a large extent on movements of K^+ across the cell membrane, between intra- and extracellular fluid. Losses of K^+ from the body (i.e. from extracellular fluid, e.g. in the urine) have only a small effect on the plasma K^+ concentration (denoted $[K^+]$), because K^+ moves out of the cells to maintain the equilibrium between intracellular and extracellular fluid. Similarly, ingestion of large amounts of K^+ has a small effect on plasma $[K^+]$ because the K^+ can enter the cells. Thus the intracellular K^+ tends to 'buffer' changes in extracellular K^+ concentration. Nevertheless, there *are* small changes in plasma $[K^+]$ when total body content of K^+ is altered.

The Body Fluid Compartments: Methods of Measurement

The volumes of several body fluid compartments can be measured using the *dilution principle*. This principle can be best illustrated by an example.

Suppose one has a bucket containing an unknown volume of water, and it is necessary to measure the volume *in situ*, i.e. without emptying the bucket — this is analogous to the measurement of a body fluid compartment. The way to determine the volume is to use a marker substance such as a dye. We can take a known quantity, Q mg, of the dye, add it to the water in the bucket, allow it to mix thoroughly so that its concentration is uniform, then take a small sample from the bucket and measure the dye concentration, C (mg/mℓ), colorimetrically. Then

$$\text{Concentration of dye } C = \frac{\text{Quantity of dye } Q \text{ (mg)}}{\text{Volume of water (m}\ell\text{)}}$$
$$\text{(mg/m}\ell\text{)}$$

$$\text{So, volume} = \frac{Q}{C}$$

It will be apparent that the measurement is valid only if the dye is uniformly mixed, and if all of it remains within the volume to be measured. In the body, the substances used to measure body fluid compartments may be excreted or metabolised, so we must modify the equation accordingly, to

$$\text{Volume of distribution} =$$
$$\frac{\text{(Quantity administered)} - \text{(Quantity metabolised or lost)}}{\text{Concentration}}$$

Almost all the substances used in measuring body fluid compartments are excreted. Some are slowly metabolised or incorporated into other

Figure 1.5: Plasma concentration of an injected amount Q, of test substance (plotted as log. conc.), as a function of time. The straight portion of the graph is extrapolated to zero time to give the plasma concentration, C, which would exist if uniform distribution could occur instantaneously. The volume of distribution is Q/C.

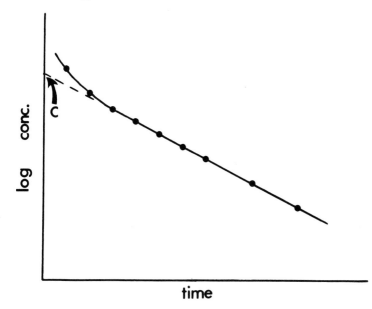

body constituents, so the above correction is usually necessary.

The test substance should ideally have the following properties:

(1) not be toxic;
(2) distribute uniformly within the compartment to be measured and not enter other compartments;
(3) not be rapidly metabolised or excreted;
(4) not alter the volume of the compartment being measured.

In practice, two variations of the dilution principle are in common use.

First, there is the single injection method. This is suitable for substances which have a slow rate of removal from the compartment being measured (by renal excretion and/or penetration into other compartments). A known amount of the test substance is injected intravenously and its plasma concentration is then determined at intervals, and a graph of concentration against time is plotted (Figure 1.5), using a log

Figure 1.6: Plasma concentration of an infused substance plotted against time. At time X, the infusion is stopped and the amount of substance excreted (Q) to reduce the plasma concentration to zero is determined. The volume of distribution is then Q/C.

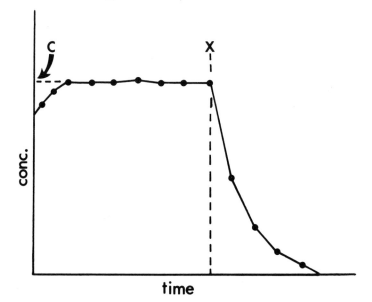

scale for the concentration axis. We can then extrapolate the straight portion of the graph back to zero time, and this gives us the plasma concentration which would have existed if the substance had instantaneously distributed itself uniformly. Dividing the amount injected by this concentration gives the compartment volume.

The second practical dilution principle method is the constant infusion method; this can be used for substances which are rapidly excreted. A loading dose of the test substance is injected to increase its plasma concentration. Then more of the test substance is infused at a rate which matches the renal excretion rate. This means that when the substance has come to equilibrium, the plasma concentration will remain constant (Figure 1.6). When this occurs, the infusion is stopped, and the urine is collected until all of the test substance is excreted. The amount excreted is then the amount which was producing the constant plasma concentration, so we can readily calculate the volume of the compartment:

$$\frac{\text{Amount excreted (mg)}}{\text{Plasma conc. (mg/\ell)}} = \text{Compartment vol. }(\ell)$$

The Measurement of Plasma Volume, Red Cell Volume and Blood Volume

For the plasma volume measurement, a substance is required which remains confined within the vascular space, i.e. does not cross the capillary endothelium. Plasma proteins are confined in this way, so radio-iodinated human serum albumin can be used, or, alternatively, a dye which binds to the plasma albumin. Such a dye is Evans blue. Since small quantities of albumin escape from the vascular system and small quantities are continually being metabolised, the plasma volume will be slightly overestimated.

When the plasma volume has been determined, the total blood volume can be readily calculated from the plasma volume and the haematocrit. The haematocrit is the percentage of total blood volume made up of red cells. It is obtained by centrifuging a small sample of blood in a closed capillary tube. Suppose the haematocrit is 45 per cent, i.e. plasma is 55 per cent of the blood volume; then

$$\text{blood volume} = \text{plasma volume} \times \frac{100}{55}$$

The normal plasma volume is 3 ℓ, and the blood volume is about 5 ℓ.

The red cell volume, although it can be calculated from the plasma volume and the haematocrit, can also be measured directly by a dilution method. A small sample of blood is taken and the red cells are incubated in a medium containing radioactive phosphorus (^{32}P) or chromium (^{51}Cr). They are then resuspended (in saline) and reinjected. After a suitable time has elapsed (e.g. 15 min) the dilution of the label is determined. (From the red cell volume and the haematocrit, the plasma volume can be calculated.)

Extracellular Fluid (ECF) Volume

The extracellular fluid volume is very difficult to determine accurately. This is because the ECF is really several compartments — plasma, interstitial fluid and transcellular fluid. The transcellular fluid is a particular problem because, as mentioned on p. 11, it is fluid separated from the plasma by another membrane in addition to the capillary endothelium; this additional membrane is normally a layer of cells. Since to measure ECF volume we need a substance which does not enter the intracellular fluid, such a substance will also not penetrate the layer of cells bounding the transcellular fluids.

The substance used to measure extracellular fluid volume must be sufficiently diffusible to cross capillary walls rapidly, so that when injected into the plasma it will enter the interstitial fluid; but it must be excluded from the cells — i.e. be unable to cross cell membranes. In fact, because different test substances fulfil these criteria to different extents, the volume of the ECF depends on the substance used to measure it.

The substances which can be used include inulin, mannitol, thiosulphate, radiosulphate, thiocyanate, radiochloride and radiosodium. Inulin (M.Wt 5,500) is the largest molecule in the group, and correspondingly has the smallest volume of distribution (approx. 12 ℓ). It may be excluded from a fraction of the interstitial fluid (e.g. in bone and cartilage). Chloride and sodium ions are not completely excluded from cells and have the largest volume of distribution (18 ℓ). Thiosulphate is probably the most widely accepted substance as a measure of extracellular fluid volume, giving a value of 15 ℓ.

Interstitial Fluid Volume

The interstitial fluid volume cannot be measured directly. It must be calculated as the difference between the extracellular fluid volume (15 ℓ measured with thiosulphate) and the plasma volume (3 ℓ) giving 12 ℓ for the interstitial fluid volume. It will be apparent, however, that the figure will depend on the substance used to measure the extracellular fluid volume.

Total Body Water

Measurement of the total body water is usually accomplished using one of the two isotopes of water (deuterium oxide or tritiated water). With either of these, we find that, in a normal 70 kg average man, about 63 per cent of the body weight is water (i.e. about 45 ℓ). In women, the proportion of the body weight which is water is only about 52 per cent. This difference, as mentioned previously, is due to the greater proportion of fat in women.

Transcellular Fluid Volume

Because the transcellular fluids are separated from the rest of the extracellular fluid by a membrane which is generally composed of intact cells, the marker substances used to measure extracellular fluid volume do not penetrate into the transcellular fluids, or do so extremely slowly. Consequently, transcellular fluid, which is included in the measurement of total body water, is generally excluded from ECF measurements. Thus,

Total body water = extracellular fluid vol. +

intracellular fluid vol. + transcellular fluid vol.

We can measure total body water and extracellular fluid volume by the dilution principle, so

Total body water − extracellular fluid vol. = intracellular

fluid vol. + transcellular fluid vol.

Although the turnover of transcellular fluid is large (up to 20 ℓ/day for the gastrointestinal tract), at any moment the absolute volume of transcellular fluid is small and is usually ignored, i.e. it is assumed that

Total body water − extracellular fluid vol. = intracellular fluid vol.

Suggestions for Further Reading

Manning, R.D. and A.C. Guyton. 'Dynamics of fluid distribution between the blood and interstitium during overhydration', *Am. J. Physiol.*, *238* (1980), pp. 645-51
Pitts, R.F. *Physiology of the Kidney and Body Fluids*, 3rd edn (Yearbook Medical Publishers, Chicago, 1974), pp. 11-35
Woodbury, D.M. 'Physiology of body fluids' in T.C. Ruch and H.D. Patton (eds), *Physiology and Biophysics*, vol. 2 (Saunders, Philadelphia, 1974), pp. 450-79

2 ESSENTIAL ANATOMY OF THE KIDNEY

Introduction

A knowledge of the structure of the kidney is essential to the understanding of its function. However, in general, structure and function are dealt with together in this book, and this chapter consists therefore of only a brief outline of those structural features which are of particular importance, or which are not dealt with in detail elsewhere.

General Morphology and Cellular Organisation

The kidneys are situated behind the peritoneum on each side of the vertebral column. In man the top (upper pole) of each kidney is at the level of the twelfth thoracic vertebra, and the bottom (lower pole) is at the level of the third lumbar vertebra. Each kidney is about 12 cm long and weighs about 150 g.

On the medial surface of each kidney (the concave surface) is a slit, the *hilus*, through which pass the renal artery and vein, the lymphatics, the renal nerve and the renal pelvis, which is the funnel-shaped upper end of the *ureter*.

The blood supply to each kidney is usually a single *renal artery* arising from the abdominal aorta. However, there may sometimes be small vessels from superior mesenteric, adrenal, spermatic or ovarian arteries.

If a kidney is bisected from top to bottom (Figure 2.1) the cut surface shows two distinct regions, a dark outer region, the cortex, and a paler inner region, the medulla, which is further divided into a number of conical areas, the renal pyramids. The apex of each pyramid extends towards the renal pelvis, forming a papilla. Some animal species have only one pyramid (and papilla) in each kidney. Striations can be seen on the renal pyramids. These are medullary rays, which are attributed to the straight tubular elements (collecting ducts and loops of Henle) and blood vessels (vasa recta) in this region.

The *renal pelvis* is lined by transitional epithelium and is the expanded upper part of the ureter. Extensions of the pelvis, the calices (sing. calyx) extend towards the papilla of each pyramid and collect the urine draining from it.

Figure 2.1: A longitudinal section of the kidney to illustrate the main structural features. The portion in the rectangle shows the arrangement of a single nephron in relation to the cortex and medulla (see also Figure 2.2). The components of the kidney are described in the text.

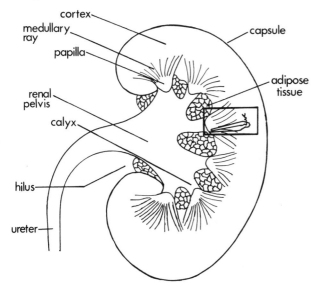

Figure 2.2: A nephron.

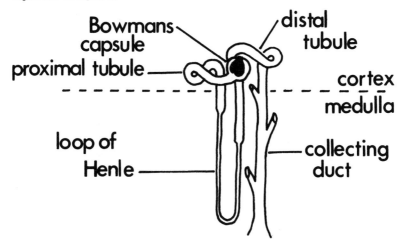

The *ureters*, about 30 cm long, are muscular tubes which connect the renal pelvis to the bladder.

The Nephron

The basic functional unit of the kidney is the nephron. Each human kidney has 1-1.5 million nephrons. The components of the nephron are shown in Figure 2.2.

The nephron is a blind-ended tube, the blind end forming a capsule (Bowman's capsule) around a knot of blood capillaries (the glomerulus). The other parts of the nephron are the proximal tubule, loop of Henle, distal tubule and collecting duct.

The glomeruli, proximal tubules and distal tubules are situated in the cortex, whereas the loops of Henle and the collecting ducts extend down through the medulla. The length of a nephron's loop of Henle depends on the location of the glomerulus, and on this basis we can identify two populations of nephrons in the human kidney (Figure 2.3).

Those nephrons with glomeruli in the outer two-thirds of the cortex are called cortical nephrons, and have very short loops of Henle, which only extend a short distance into the medulla (or, indeed, may not reach the medulla at all). In contrast, nephrons whose glomeruli are in the inner one-third of the cortex (juxtamedullary nephrons) have long loops of Henle which pass deeply into the medulla. In man about 15 per cent of nephrons are long-looped. (The proportion of long-looped nephrons is different in different species, e.g. in the rat the figure is 30 per cent.)

The Glomerulus

The function of the glomerulus is to produce an ultrafiltrate of plasma, which enters the nephrons (see Chapter 3). In man, the glomerulus has a diameter of about 200 μm. Each glomerulus is supplied with blood by an *afferent* arteriole, which divides within the glomerulus to form the tuft of glomerular capillaries. These capillaries rejoin to form the *efferent* arteriole. Details of glomerular structure are given in Chapter 3.

Proximal Tubules

The proximal tubule is the first segment of the nephron after the Bowman's capsule; its initial segment (pars convoluta) is convoluted, but further along it becomes straight (pars recta) and passes down towards the medulla where it becomes the descending limb of the loop of Henle. The length of a human proximal tubule is generally about

Figure 2.3: Cortical (short-looped) and juxtamedullary (long-looped) nephrons, showing the differences in the blood supply to the two nephron types.

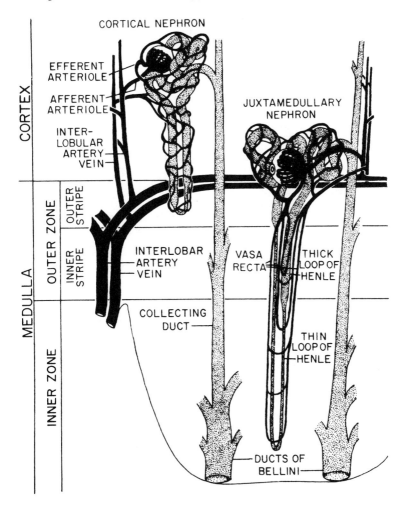

Source: Reproduced with permission from Pitts, R.F. *Physiology of the Kidney and Body Fluids*, 3rd edn (Year Book Medical Publishers, Chicago, 1974).

15 mm (12-25 mm range) with a diameter (outside) of 70 μm.

The convoluted segment of the proximal tubule consists of cuboidal/columnar cells, which on their luminal surface have a 'brush border'. This consists of millions of microvilli with a density of about 150 per

Figure 2.4: The morphology of proximal tubule cells. Above: a cell in the pars convoluta. These cells have numerous microvilli on the luminal surface, forming a 'brush border'. The peritubular surface of the cell has basal infoldings and rests on a basement membrane. There are numerous mitochondria, suggesting that the cells have high energy consumption (for active transport). Below: a cell in the pars recta. There are fewer mitochondria and fewer microvilli, suggesting that the transport functions of the cells are less well developed than those of pars convoluta cells.

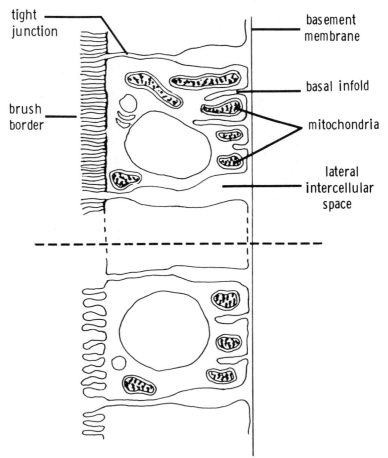

cubic micron of cell surface. This brush border increases tremendously the surface area available for the absorption of tubular fluid. Adjacent cells are joined tightly together close to their luminal surface (at a 'tight junction' or zonula occludens), but on the peritubular side of the tight junction there is a space between adjacent cells, the lateral intercellular space (Figure 2.4).

The cells of the straight part of the proximal tubule, the pars recta (which can also be regarded as the beginning of the loop of Henle), are very similar to those of the convoluted segment, but have a less dense brush border (i.e. fewer microvilli), contain fewer mitochondria and are generally more flattened.

Loop of Henle

The loop of Henle is generally considered to begin at the transition from thick-walled tubule to thin-walled tubule (Figure 2.2). The cells of the thin part of the loop of Henle are squamous, i.e. are very thin and flattened. Under the light microscope, the cells of the loop of Henle resemble capillary endothelial cells; however, under the electron microscope, significant differences are apparent. The contours of the cells are extremely complex, the cells interdigitate with their neighbours and there are a few microvilli on the luminal cell surfaces.

The cells of the thin ascending limb of the loop of Henle are structurally similar to those of the descending limb, but there may be important functional differences (see p. 67), particularly in their permeability properties (and possibly in their capability for active transport). The thin segment of the loop is up to 15 mm long, and the external diameter is about 20 μm. The thick ascending segment of the loop of Henle is a cuboidal/columnar epithelium, with cells of a similar size to those in the proximal tubule. However, the cells do not have a brush border like that of the proximal tubule, and although there are many infoldings and projections of the cell on the luminal surface, there are fewer basal infoldings. This portion of the nephron continues into the cortex as the distal tubule. However, the term 'distal' tubule is a purely *anatomical* description of the location of a portion of the nephron, and has no *functional* meaning. Functionally, the thick ascending limb of the loop of Henle meets the cortical collecting ducts. In the region where the ascending limb of the loop enters the cortex, it is closely associated with the glomerulus and afferent arteriole, and consists of modified *macula densa* cells (see p. 39).

Collecting Duct

Most of the cells in the collecting duct are cuboidal, with a much less granular cytoplasm than that of the proximal tubule cells and only a few corrugations on the luminal surface. Interspersed with the cells of this type, there are a few cells having more granular cytoplasm.

In the cortex, each collecting duct receives about six 'distal tubules', and as the ducts enter the medulla, they join with each other in successive pairings to form a duct of Bellini up to 200 μm wide, which drains into a renal calyx. Strictly speaking, anatomically the 'nephron' does not include the collecting duct (and is embryologically distinct from it). However, functionally the collecting duct is an essential part of the nephron unit.

Blood Supply and Vascular Structure within the Kidney

The kidneys have a high blood flow, receiving between them a little over 20 per cent of the cardiac output. (This is about five times the flow to exercising skeletal muscle, and almost ten times the coronary blood flow, on the basis of flow per unit tissue weight.)

Figure 2.5: A longitudinal section of the kidney, showing the arrangement of the major blood vessels.

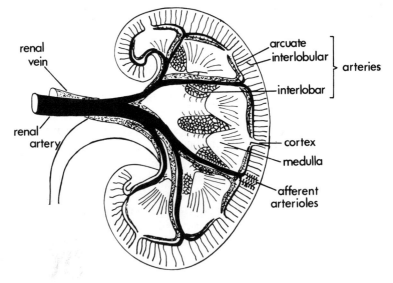

Almost all of the blood which enters the kidneys does so at the renal hilus, via the *renal artery*. The renal artery branches (Figure 2.5) to form several *interlobar arteries*, which themselves branch to give rise to *arcuate* (or arciform) *arteries*, which pass along the boundary between cortex and medulla. From the arcuate arteries, branches travel out at right angles, through the cortex towards the capsule. These are *interlobular arteries*, and the *afferent arterioles* which supply the glomerular capillaries branch off from the interlobular arteries.

The glomerular capillaries are the site of filtration of the blood, the filtrate entering the Bowman's capsule of the nephron. The glomerular capillaries do not drain into a vein; instead they drain into a second arteriole, the *efferent arteriole*. (The efferent arterioles can be regarded as portal blood vessels. Portal vessels carry blood from a capillary network directly to a second capillary network.)

The efferent arterioles from nephrons in the outer two-thirds of the cortex branch to form a dense network of *peritubular capillaries*, which surround all the cortical tubular elements. The efferent arterioles in the inner one-third of the cortex give rise to some peritubular capillaries, but also give rise to capillaries which have a hairpin course into and out of the medulla, where they are adjacent to the loops of Henle and collecting tubules. These medullary capillaries are *vasa recta* (Figure 2.3). Vasa recta and peritubular capillaries eventually drain into the renal vein which leaves the kidney at the hilus.

Most of the renal blood flow (more than 90 per cent) goes to the renal cortex, which is perfused at a rate of about 500 ml/min/100 g tissue. The outer medulla has a much lower flow (100 ml/min/100 g tissue), and the inner medulla has an extremely low flow (20 ml/min/100 g tissue).

The Function of the Renal Blood Supply

In most organs and tissues of the body, the main purpose of the blood supply is to provide oxygen and remove carbon dioxide and other products of metabolism. The renal cortex receives far more oxygen than it requires, so that the arteriovenous O_2 difference is only 1-2 per cent. This is because the high renal blood supply exists to maintain a high glomerular filtration rate. Surprisingly (at first sight), if the renal blood supply is reduced, the arteriovenous O_2 difference generally does not increase. This is because the blood flow determines the rate of filtration, and more than 50 per cent of the O_2 consumption is used for sodium reabsorption (see Chapter 3). So if filtration rate is reduced reabsorption can occur at a lower rate and O_2 consumption is also reduced. The control of the renal blood supply is considered later (Chapter 6).

In spite of the very high blood flow to the kidneys, the medullary blood supply is no more than adequate for the supply of oxygen to medullary cells, because the vasa recta arrangement causes oxygen to short-circuit the loops of Henle (see p. 74).

The Renal Lymphatic Drainage

Renal lymph vessels begin as blind-ended tubes in the renal cortex (close to the corticomedullary junction), and run parallel to the arcuate veins to leave the kidney at the renal hilus. Other lymph vessels travel towards the cortex and may pass through the capsule. The importance of the renal lymphatic drainage is frequently overlooked, but in fact the volume of lymph draining into the renal hilus per minute is about 0.5 mℓ (i.e. the kidney produces almost as much lymph per minute as urine). Its function is probably to return protein reabsorbed from the tubular fluid, to the blood.

Figure 2.6: The juxtaglomerular apparatus. The beginning of the distal tubule (i.e. where the loop of Henle re-enters the cortex) lies very close to the afferent and efferent arterioles, and the cells of both the afferent arterioles and the tubule show specialisation. The cells of the afferent arteriole wall are thickened, granular juxtaglomerular cells. The cells in the tubule form the macula densa.

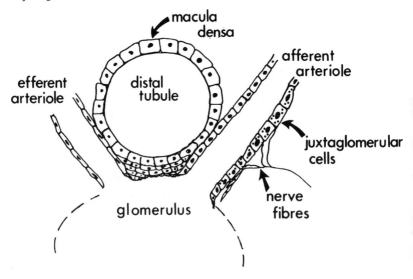

The Juxtaglomerular Apparatus

The ascending limb of the loop of Henle, where it re-enters the cortex and becomes the distal tubule, passes very close to the Bowman's capsule of its own nephron, and comes into contact with the afferent and efferent arterioles from its own glomerulus (Figure 2.6). In this area of close association between the distal tubule and the arterioles is the juxtaglomerular apparatus; it consists of specialised structures in the walls of the afferent arteriole and of the distal tubule. The specialised cells in the distal tubule are *macula densa* cells. They respond to the composition of the fluid within the tubule (see p. 101). The specialised cells in the afferent arteriolar wall are *granular cells*. They release the enzyme (hormone) *renin*. The control of the release of renin, and its actions, are the subject of a later section (Chapter 8).

The cells of the juxtaglomerular apparatus are modified smooth muscle cells. The granules in the granular cells contain stored renin, and it is likely that the non-granular cells of the juxtaglomerular area are capable of becoming granular cells and of releasing renin.

Suggestions for Further Reading

Maunsbach, A.B. 'Ultrastructure of the proximal tubule' in J. Orloff and R.W. Berliner (eds), *Handbook of Physiology, Section 8, Renal Physiology* (American Physiological Society, Washington, 1973), pp. 31-79
Osvaldo-Decima, L. 'Ultrastructure of the lower nephron' in ibid., pp. 81-102

3 GLOMERULAR FILTRATION

The Filter

Urine is initially an ultrafiltrate of the plasma. Ultrafiltration occurs from the glomerulus (a tuft of capillaries) into the Bowman's capsule (the blind end of a nephron) — see Figure 3.1. In moving from the capillary into the Bowman's capsule, the filtrate must traverse three layers. These are:

(1) the endothelial cell lining of the glomerular capillaries;
(2) the glomeruluar basement membrane (non-cellular — composed of connective tissues);
(3) the visceral epithelial cells of the Bowman's capsule.

Since the properties of the glomerular filter are dependent on these structures, we will begin by looking in more detail at the morphology of the glomerulus and Bowman's capsule.

Figure 3.2 shows diagrammatically the arrangement of the cellular elements of the glomerulus, and in Figure 3.3 there are electron micrographs showing the true arrangement of the glomerular components. The endothelial cells which form the glomerular capillaries have thin, flattened cytoplasmic areas, but the nuclei are large, may be folded or distorted, and bulge out into the capillary lumen. There are few mitochondria in these cells. Adjacent cells are in contact with each other, but the contact appears to be incomplete. However, there is some controversy about whether the 'gaps' are in fact fenestrations (holes), or whether they are areas where the cytoplasm of the endothelial cells is very thin.

Immediately beneath the endothelial cells is a basement membrane; it forms a continuous layer, and is thought to be the main barrier to the filtration of large molecules. It consists of collagen (or a collagen-like protein) and other glycoproteins.

The third layer of the filter consists of the visceral epithelial cells of Bowman's capsule. These cells are called podocytes and have an extremely complex morphology. The cell body has projections from it (trabeculae) which encircle the basement membrane around the capillary. From the trabeculae project many smaller processes (pedicels). The pedicels interdigitate with those of adjacent trabeculae, and it is

40

Figure 3.1: Diagrammatic representation of the glomerulus and Bowman's capsule. Bowman's capsule is the blind end of the nephron and is invaginated by the capillary loops of the glomerulus. The figure is diagrammatic rather than anatomically accurate, in several respects. In reality, the afferent arteriole, as it enters Bowman's capsule, branches to form about six vessels. Each of these subdivides to form a knot of about 40 glomerular capillary loops, and there are many interconnections between these capillary loops. The epithelium of Bowman's capsule in contact with the capillaries is a highly specialised cell layer – the podocytes. This is shown in the diagram as covering only a small area of the capillaries, whereas in reality it covers the entire surface of the glomerular blood vessels. A way of envisaging this is to think of the Bowman's capsule as a balloon. The capillaries pressed into the 'balloon' will be covered completely by it. The basement membrane of the outer part of Bowman's capsule is continuous with the basement membrane of the rest of the nephron, and is also present between the capillary endothelium and the podocytes (see Figure 3.2).

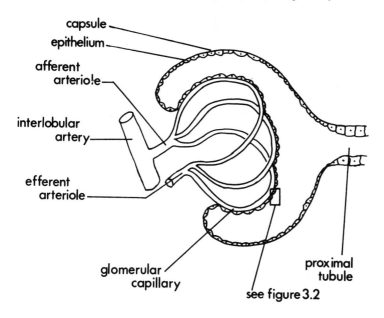

thought that in living animals the pedicels are in contact with each other (although after fixation for microscopy, gaps appear to be present); this contact means that substances passing through the slits (slit pores) between adjacent pedicels must pass through the surface coating of the pedicels (the 'slit diaphragm'), and this influences the filtration behaviour of large, charged molecules (see below). Although at various times special filtration functions have been attributed to the podocytes, it seems likely that the main function of these cells is to lay down and

Figure 3.2: The arrangement of the elements of the glomerulus through which the filtrate must pass to enter the nephron.

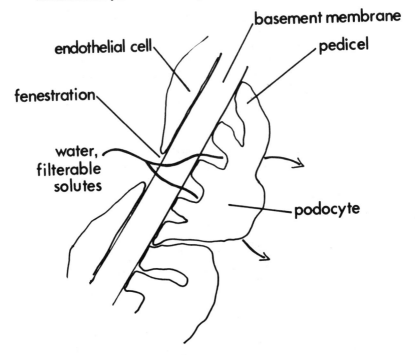

maintain the basement membrane.

Mesangial Cells

In the central part of the glomerular tuft there are a number of irregularly shaped cells, termed mesangial cells. These are actively phagocytic and may prevent the accumulation in the basement membrane of macromolecules which have escaped from the capillaries. The cells may also have a structural role in holding the delicate glomerular structure in position, and in addition are capable of contraction (i.e. behave like smooth muscle cells).

The Glomerular Filtration Process

An almost protein-free ultrafiltrate passes into Bowman's capsule from the glomerular capillaries. Molecular size is the main determinant of whether a substance will be filtered or will be retained in the capillaries.

Figure 3.3: (a) Scanning electron micrograph (× 2,000 approximately) of part of a glomerulus from a normal rat kidney. The visceral epithelial cells or podocytes (P) have many processes or trabeculae (I) extending from the cell body, and wrapping around the glomerular capillaries. From the trabeculae extend many hundreds of smaller processes, the foot processes or pedicels, which interdigitate with each other and completely cover the capillary surfaces. Note that the interdigitating foot processes arise from different podocytes. (b) Electron micrograph (× 75,000 approximately) of normal rat glomerulus. CL – capillary lumen; BS – Bowman's space (i.e. within Bowman's capsule); P – Pedicels embedded in the basement membrane (broad arrow). The thin arrow shows a 'filtration slit', between adjacent pedicels. This is probably a fixation artifact, with the pedicels in contact with each other during life. Note the apparent gaps in the capillary endothelial layer. The dark mass in the lower right of the picture is an erythrocyte.

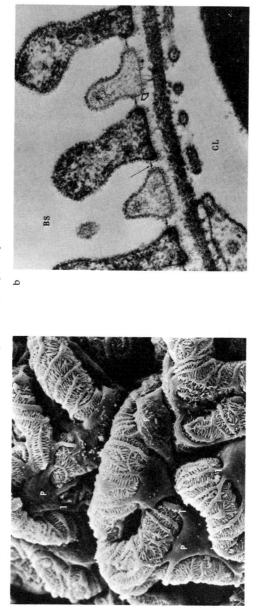

b

a

Source: Reproduced with permission from Brenner, B.M. and Rector, F.C. (eds), *The Kidney*, vol. 1 (Saunders, Philadelphia, 1976).

Figure 3.4: The filtration properties of the glomerular filter. The solid line shows the filtrate/plasma ratio (F/P ratio) for substances which occur naturally in the body. For substances up to molecular weight 7,000, the filter permits free filtration, i.e. solutes pass through as readily as the solvent (H_2O), and the filtrate/plasma ratio is 1. Higher molecular weight molecules (proteins) are retarded by the filter, so the filtrate/plasma ratio is less than 1. Filtration of molecules with a molecular weight of 70,000 and above is insignificant. Molecular charge, as well as molecular size, determines the filtration of large molecules. The dotted line shows the filtrate/plasma ratio of uncharged dextran molecules. They are filtered to a greater extent than are (negatively charged) protein molecules of the same molecular weight.

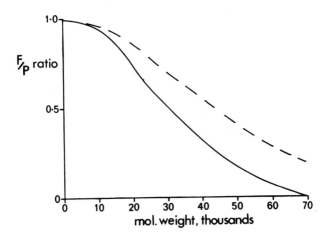

However, molecular shape and charge also influence the filtration process, though these factors are of significance only for large molecules. For example, the rate of filtration of albumin (M.Wt 69,000), which has a negative charge, is only about one-twentieth that of uncharged dextran molecules of the same molecular weight (Figure 3.4). This finding suggests that the glomerular filtration barrier (the basement membrane and the pedicels) has fixed anions, which repel anionic macromolecules and thereby hinder or prevent the filtration of such molecules.

What exactly is meant by the term 'filtration' (or ultrafiltration)? Filtration is the *bulk flow* of solvent through a filter, carrying with it those solutes which are small enough to pass through the filter. The prefix 'ultra' simply means that the filter operates at the molecular level (in contrast to the macroscopic particle level of conventional filters).

In the glomerulus, the molecular-weight cut-off for the filter is about 70,000. Plasma albumin, with a molecular weight of 69,000, passes through the filter in minute quantities (retarded also by its charge, as mentioned above). Smaller molecules pass through the filter more easily, but the filter is freely permeable only to those molecules with a molecular weight less than about 7,000. The relationship between molecular weight and filtration characteristics is shown in Figure 3.4.

Since the glomerular filter permits the free passage of molecules of molecular weight less than 7,000, the initial glomerular filtrate will contain small molecules and ions (e.g. glucose, amino acids, urea, sodium, potassium) in almost exactly the same concentrations as the afferent arteriolar concentrations, and similarly the efferent arteriolar concentrations of such substances will not have been significantly altered by the filtration process. (There will be very small concentration differences due to the Gibbs-Donnan effect across the glomerular capillary membrane.)

In man, the glomerular filtration rate (GFR) is about 180 ℓ/day (125 mℓ/min). Since the filtrate is derived from plasma, and the average person has only 3 ℓ of plasma, it follows that this same plasma is filtered (and reabsorbed in the tubules) many times in the course of a day. Yet, despite the magnitude of glomerular filtration, the forces determining filtration are not fundamentally different in nature from those forces determining the formation of tissue fluid through capillaries elsewhere in the body, and it is of interest to consider the process of tissue fluid formation and reabsorption in ordinary capillaries, before considering the special case of the glomerular capillaries.

Vascular beds, in any tissue, consist of a set of different kinds of vessels, connected in series. In typical systemic vascular beds, e.g. in skin or muscle, the vessels are: arterioles, capillaries, venules and veins.

The pressure drop along an idealised capillary from the arteriolar end to the venous end is shown in Figure 3.5. At the arteriolar end, the forces causing fluid to leave the capillary and enter the interstitial fluid are greater than the forces tending to retain fluid in the capillary and so tissue fluid formation occurs. In contrast, at the venous end of the capillary, the forces leading to the re-entry of fluid into the capillaries exceed those forcing fluid out, and tissue fluid reabsorption occurs. Consequently, there is a balance between formation and reabsorption of tissue fluid.

In the glomerular capillaries, the anatomical arrangement of the blood vessels alters the magnitude of the forces causing fluid

Figure 3.5: The fall in mean blood pressure from arteries to capillaries in a typical systemic vascular bed (e.g. in muscle). The main resistance to flow, and hence the biggest pressure drop, is in the arterioles. The plasma protein osmotic pressure (oncotic pressure) in the capillaries (Π_{cap}) is normally 25 mm Hg. In the region 'a' of the capillaries, the hydrostatic pressure exceeds the plasma protein osmotic pressure, and there is net fluid movement out of the capillary. In the region 'b', the pressure gradient is reversed, and there is net fluid movement into the capillary. (Only the capillaries have highly permeable walls, and hence it is only in the capillaries that the plasma-interstitial fluid pressure gradients determine fluid movements.)

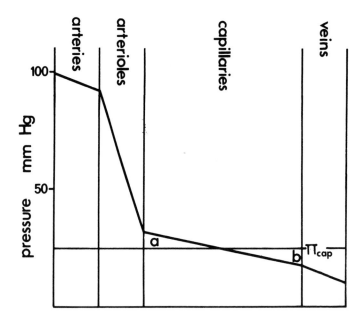

movements across the capillaries, as shown in Figure 3.6. The sequence of blood vessels is: afferent arterioles, glomerular capillaries, efferent arterioles, peritubular capillaries, venules and veins. The presence of a second resistance vessel, the efferent arteriole, means that the hydrostatic pressure in the glomerular capillaries falls very little throughout their length. This pressure is slightly higher, at 45 mm Hg, than that in the capillaries of most other vascular beds (about 32 mm Hg). This does not, however, mean that filtration out of the glomerular capillaries occurs along their entire length, because, as the filtration process occurs, the non-filterable substances (including the plasma proteins) become progressively more concentrated. Thus the oncotic pressure in the capillaries increases and eventually, when oncotic pressure reaches

Figure 3.6: The pressure in the blood vessels of the glomerulus, showing the forces for fluid movement across the glomerular capillary. By comparison with Figure 3.5, it can be seen that the pressure falls less along the renal afferent arterioles than in muscle arterioles (to 45 mm Hg instead of 32 mm Hg), and the pressure in the glomerular capillaries (P_{cap}) is maintained and falls very little along the length of the capillary. This is because of the resistance vessel beyond the capillary, the efferent arteriole. The pressure P_{cap} (45 mm Hg) is a force for the formation of glomerular filtrate. This force is opposed by the hydrostatic pressure in the Bowman's capsule (P_{bc}), normally 10 mm Hg, and by the plasma protein osmotic pressure (oncotic pressure) in the capillaries, Π_{cap}, which is initially 25 mm Hg, but as filtration proceeds the plasma proteins in the capillary become progressively more concentrated and so Π_{cap} increases. Eventually the forces opposing filtration ($\Pi_{cap} + P_{bc}$) equal the force favouring filtration, and net filtration ceases. This balance is normally achieved well before the end of the glomerular capillary.

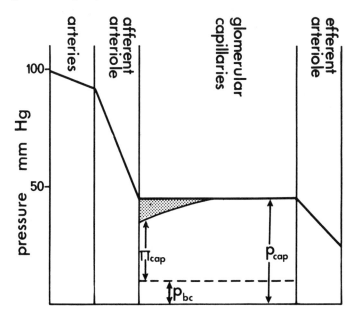

about 35 mm Hg, the net ultrafiltration pressure has been reduced to zero. For further explanation, see legend to Figure 3.6.

The forces governing glomerular filtration are called Starling's forces, i.e. hydrostatic pressure gradients and oncotic pressure gradients. Putting this into a mathematical formulation, we can say that

GFR $\propto$ Forces favouring filtration $-$ forces opposing filtration

$$\propto (P_{cap} + \Pi_{bc}) - (P_{bc} + \Pi_{cap})$$

where P_{cap} is glomerular capillary hydrostatic pressure, Π_{bc} is the oncotic pressure in Bowman's capsule, P_{bc} is the hydrostatic pressure in Bowman's capsule and Π_{cap} is the oncotic pressure in the glomerular capillaries. Since negligible amounts of protein enter the Bowman's capsule, Π_{bc} is normally zero, and

$$\text{GFR} \propto P_{cap} - P_{bc} - \Pi_{cap}$$

P_{bc} is usually about 10 mm Hg, and Π_{cap} changes as filtration proceeds, as described above.

Glomerular Capillary Permeability

In order to convert the above equation for GFR into real measurements we have to introduce a term (K_f) for the capillary permeability and the area of capillary available for filtration, i.e.

$$\text{GFR} = K_f \left(P_{cap} - P_{bc} - \Pi_{cap} \right)$$

The permeability of glomerular capillaries is about 100 times greater than the permeability of capillaries elsewhere in the body.

The Physiological Regulation of GFR

When the mean renal arterial pressure is within the range 90-190 mm Hg, changes in arterial pressure do not generally lead to changes in GFR. This is true both in intact kidneys, in denervated kidneys and in isolated, perfused kidneys. Because the ability to maintain a constant GFR resides within the kidney itself, the process is called *autoregulation*. Autoregulation of renal blood flow also occurs and the phenomenon will be considered further in Chapter 6.

The Composition of the Glomerular Filtrate

Table 3.1 shows the plasma and Bowman's capsular concentrations of some major solutes. The normal urinary concentrations are also shown. It can be seen that, whereas the filtration process produces no significant changes in the concentrations of small solutes, the tubular fluid has been considerably modified by the time it is excreted. These modifications to the filtrate, which occur in the rest of the nephron, will be considered in the next two chapters.

Although the quantity of protein filtered at the glomerulus is

Table 3.1: Normal solute concentrations in plasma, plasma water, the initial ultrafiltrate in Bowman's capsule and the final urine. The differences in solute concentrations between Bowman's capsule fluid and the plasma water are caused by Gibbs-Donnan effects (see Chapter 1). The figures for the urinary concentrations of electrolytes are typical values; wider variations are possible.

	Plasma (mmol/ℓ)	Plasma Water (mmol/ℓ)	Bowman's Capsule (mmol/ℓ)	Urine (mmol/ℓ)
Sodium	142	153	142	50–150
Potassium	4.0	4.3	4.0	20–100
Chloride	103	109	113	50–150
Bicarbonate	24–27	26–29	27–30	0–25
Glucose	5.5	5.9	5.9	0
Protein	6 g/100 mℓ	–	0.020 g/100 mℓ	<0.010 g/100 mℓ

small, its loss in the urine would represent a considerable wastage over the course of a day. Most of the filtered protein is reabsorbed in the proximal tubule and enters the renal lymph vessels. The amount of protein entering the renal lymph vessels per day is about 30 g, which is equal to the amount of protein entering the glomerular filtrate, i.e. essentially *all* of the filtered protein is reabsorbed into the renal lymph vessels.

The Filtration Fraction

The renal blood flow is large in relation to the size of the kidneys (about 1.1 ℓ/min), but only a relatively small fraction of this is filtered. In fact, since a proportion of the blood is cells (which are not filterable), the *renal plasma flow* is the amount of fluid entering the kidney which is potentially filterable. The renal plasma flow is about 600 mℓ/min.

The normal glomerular filtration rate is 125 mℓ/min. Thus the *filtration fraction* is 125/600 or approximately 20 per cent, i.e. of every 600 mℓ of plasma arriving at the glomeruli, about 475 mℓ continues into the efferent arerioles.

The Glomerular Filtration Pressure as a Force for Tubular Flow

The net filtration pressure must be sufficient to move plasma out of the glomerular capillary and into the Bowman's capsule, but in addition, it must also maintain the flow of fluid along the nephron. The pressure in the Bowman's capsule (P_{bc}) must therefore be high

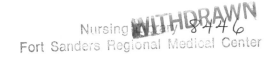

enough to overcome the viscosity of the tubular fluid and its friction against the tubule walls, and to maintain the tubules in a patent form, against the renal interstitial pressure tending to compress the tubules. Occlusion of the renal blood supply, so that filtration ceases, causes the collapse of the tubular lumens.

Suggestions for Further Reading

Brenner, B.M. and W.M. Deen. 'The physiological basis of glomerular ultrafiltration' in K. Thurau (ed.), *Kidney and Urinary Tract Physiology*, MTP International Review of Science, Physiology Series 1, vol. 6 (Butterworths, London, 1974), pp. 335-56

Brenner, B.M., T.H. Hostetter and H.D. Humes. 'Glomerular permselectivity: barrier function based on discrimination of molecular size and charge', *Am. J. Physiol., 234* (1978), pp. F455-60

Farquhar, M.G. 'The primary glomerular filtration barrier: basement membrane or epithelial slits?', *Kidney Int., 8* (1975), pp. 197-211

Michael, A.F., W.F. Keane, L. Raij, R.L. Vernier and S.M. Mauer. 'The glomerular mesangium', *Kidney Int., 17* (1980), pp. 141-54

4 THE PROXIMAL TUBULE

General Principles of Tubular Function

The fluid entering the proximal tubule from the glomerulus has a composition very similar to that of plasma, except that plasma proteins, which cannot readily cross the filtration barrier, are almost completely absent from the tubular fluid. In the proximal tubule, 60-70 per cent of the filtrate is *reabsorbed*; some ions and molecules, however, are *secreted*.

In the kidney tubules, the terms 'reabsorption' and 'secretion' indicate the direction of movement; reabsorption is movement of a substance from the tubular fluid into the tubule cells (and thence into the blood), whereas secretion is movement from the tubule cells into the tubular fluid. Neither term conveys any information about the nature of the forces causing the movement, which may be either active or passive. In Chapter 1, we saw that active transport is important in enabling cells to maintain their normal ionic composition and volume. In the kidney, active transport processes not only serve this purpose, but also make possible the movement of substances right through cells — i.e. from the tubular lumen to the peritubular side, or vice versa.

The single most important event in the proximal tubule is the reabsorption of 60-70 per cent of the filtered sodium, by an active (i.e. energy-consuming) process, which accounts for much of the oxygen consumption of the kidney. In order to understand it, a knowledge of the proximal tubular structure is necessary.

The morphology of the proximal tubule cells was covered briefly in Chapter 2, but will be considered in more detail here. The proximal tubule is divisible into the convoluted portion, or pars convoluta, which begins immediately behind the glomerulus, and the straight portion, or pars recta, which passes into the medulla to become the loop of Henle. The cells of these two portions have somewhat different structures (Figure 2.4) and there are cells of an intermediate type linking the two portions. The transport functions of the proximal tubule are primarily dependent on the pars convoluta cells.

Adjacent proximal tubule cells are in close contact with each other at the luminal side (the tight junction), but there are gaps between the cells — lateral intercellular spaces — at the peritubular side. The

51

luminal surface has a brush border of microvilli, which greatly increases the surface area available for absorption (Figure 2.4).

Proximal Tubular Handling of Sodium

The reabsorption of sodium is of great significance, not only because of the importance of sodium to the body, but also because the reabsorption processes for many other substances (including chloride, water, glucose and amino acids) are dependent on sodium reabsorption.

Figure 4.1: Sodium chloride and water movements across proximal tubule cells. The tubular lumen is on the left and the peritubular capillary on the right. Passive movements are shown as dotted lines, active movements as solid lines. The Na^+ concentration in the tubular lumen (and in the peritubular capillary) is 140 mM, whereas inside the tubule cell it is only about 30 mM. Hence passive sodium entry is favoured by both concentration and electrical gradients. Cl^- passively follows Na^+ to maintain electrical neutrality. There is also some active H^+ secretion from cell to lumen (see Figure 4.7). Active Na^+ extrusion from the cell occurs at the peritubular side. Much of this active transport is directed into the lateral intercellular spaces. Some of this transport is via a Na^+-K^+ ATPase, but there may also be K^+- independent Na^+ extrusion. Cl^- follows sodium into the lateral intercellular spaces along the electrical gradient, and water accompanies the NaCl osmotically. Some of the NaCl and water which enters the lateral intercellular spaces re-enters the tubular lumen by passing through the 'tight' junctions.

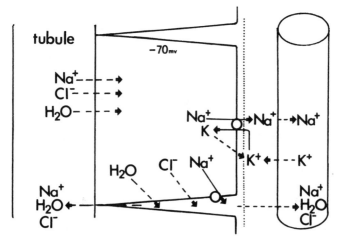

The proximal tubule is highly permeable to sodium in both directions; net reabsorption from the tubule is the result of slightly greater efflux from the lumen than influx into it, and in fact net sodium entry into the peritubular capillaries is only about 20 per cent of the unidirectional sodium efflux from the tubular lumen, because there is a high backflux. Whereas the efflux from the lumen occurs mainly *through* the cells, much of the backflux is via intercellular channels – i.e. *between* the cells (Figure 4.1).

Sodium Entry

The proximal tubule cells have a negative intracellular potential of approximately −70 mV relative to both luminal fluid and peritubular fluid, and the cells also have a low intracellular sodium concentration (less than 30 mM). So sodium movement from the luminal fluid into the cell is down a large electrical gradient and also down a chemical concentration gradient; thus sodium entry into the cell occurs passively. However, there is evidence that this entry of sodium into the cells is the rate-limiting step in the transfer process.

Sodium Extrusion

Sodium extrusion from the tubular cells occurs against electrical and chemical gradients, and is accompanied by the entry into the cells of potassium ions. Since ATP is converted to ADP to provide energy for the transport, the transport mechanism is termed an Na^+-K^+-ATPase. This process has little effect on the intracellular K^+ concentration, since K^+ can readily cross cell membranes and so rapidly diffuses out of the cells. The ratio of transport is not 1:1 (in fact more sodium leaves than K^+ enters). It is thought that there may also be a sodium-extruding pump which is not an Na^+-K^+-ATPase (Figure 4.1).

The active extrusion of sodium from the tubule cells occurs almost entirely across the basolateral surfaces of the cells, and much of this transport is directed into the lateral intercellular spaces. The significance of this will be clear later.

Chloride Reabsorption

There is a large (70 mV) electrical gradient opposing chloride entry into the cells from the lumen. It is possible that there is a 'co-transport' mechanism, whereby the passive entry of sodium into the cell facilitates the entry of chloride (see also the sections on glucose and amino acid absorption). Chloride leaves the cells passively to enter the lateral intercellular spaces along with sodium.

Water Reabsorption

The active extrusion of Na^+ from the tubular cells into lateral inter-cellular spaces, accompanied passively by Cl^-, leads to the accumulation of NaCl in the spaces and hence a local increase in osmotic pressure, which causes osmotic entry of water into the spaces via the cells.

Uptake of NaCl and Water into Peritubular Capillaries

The end result of the processes described so far is the entry of isotonic NaCl solution (from the tubule) into the lateral intercellular spaces. From here, the NaCl solution can move in two possible directions: (1) into the capillaries or (2) back into the tubular lumen through the tight junction.

A proportion of the NaCl always leaks back, and hence the sodium reabsorption process can be called a 'pump-leak' system (it is also known as a gradient-time limited transport process). It is likely that alterations in the rate of proximal tubular sodium reabsorption are brought about by changes in the rate of backflux (from the lateral intercellular spaces) into the tubule, and not by changes in the rate of active sodium extrusion from the cells.

Changes in the rate of backflux occur as a result of changes in the rate of uptake from the lateral intercellular spaces into the capillaries. The faster the capillary uptake the lower the rate of backflux will be (Figure 4.2). What then determines the rate at which sodium chloride solution is transferred from the lateral intercellular spaces into the capillaries?

The forces governing the movement of fluid across the walls of the peritubular capillaries are Starling forces – i.e. oncotic pressure and hydrostatic pressure gradients. So capillary uptake from the lateral intercellular spaces is determined as follows:

Capillary uptake $\propto$ forces favouring uptake – forces opposing uptake

$$\propto (\Pi_{cap} + P_{LIS}) - (\Pi_{LIS} + P_{cap})$$

where Π_{cap} and Π_{LIS} are oncotic pressures in the peritubular capillary

Figure 4.2: The uptake of sodium, chloride and water from the lateral intercellular spaces into the peritubular capillaries, showing the forces involved (Starling forces). The only active process is sodium extrusion from the cell into the lateral intercellular space. Cl^- and H_2O follow passively along electrical and osmotic gradients, respectively. The solution (H_2O containing Na^+ and Cl^-) in the lateral intercellular space can move into the capillary, or leak back into the tubular lumen through the 'tight' junction. The forces favouring uptake into the capillary are the oncotic pressure in the capillary (Π_{cap}) and the hydrostatic pressure in the lateral intercellular space (P_{LIS}). The forces opposing uptake are the capillary hydrostatic pressure (P_{cap}) and the lateral intercellular space oncotic pressure (Π_{LIS}). It is thought that the rate of active transport of Na^+ into the lateral intercellular space is relatively constant, and changes in proximal tubular NaCl and water reabsorption are due to changes in the rate of capillary uptake and backflux.

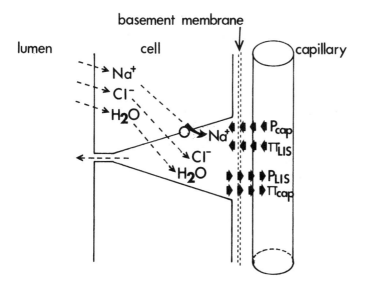

and the lateral intercellular space respectively (the latter is normally negligible) and P_{cap} and P_{LIS} are the hydrostatic pressures in the capillary and the lateral intercellular space. The forces are shown diagrammatically in Figure 4.2.

Relationship of Proximal Tubular Reabsorption to Glomerular Filtration Rate

It is important at this stage to bear in mind that the peritubular capillaries are branches of the efferent arterioles, which in turn arise from the glomerular capillaries. Consequently, the Starling forces in the peritubular capillaries can be modified by the glomerular filtration process.

The peritubular capillary oncotic pressure (Π_{cap}) is determined by the plasma protein concentration. Since the plasma proteins are concentrated in the glomerular capillaries by the filtration process, Π_{cap} will depend partly on the filtration fraction (GFR/RPF, see p. 49 and 84).

The peritubular capillary hydrostatic pressure will be determined mainly by the venous pressure (see p. 152), but it is possible that changes in the degree to which arterial pressure is transmitted to the capillaries (via afferent and efferent arterioles) can also determine P_{cap}.

The dependence of Π_{cap} on the filtration fraction provides a mechanism whereby proximal tubular reabsorption can be adjusted automatically to compensate for changes in glomerular filtration — thus if GFR increases, the forces available to reabsorb the increased volume of filtrate also increase, automatically. Thus there is *glomerulo-tubular balance*, whereby an essentially fixed percentage of the glomerular filtrate will be reabsorbed proximally, i.e. there is normally a relatively constant proximal tubular fractional reabsorption.

However, proximal tubular fractional reabsorption can be altered, e.g. by alterations in the effective circulating volume. Such alterations are considered later (pp. 104-5).

Proximal Tubular Reabsorption of Other Solutes

The importance of sodium reabsorption in the proximal tubule derives not only from the necessity of conserving filtered sodium, but also from the effects of sodium reabsorption on the reabsorption of other solutes.

Sodium reabsorption leads to electrical, concentration and osmotic gradients for the passive reabsorption of such solutes as chloride, potassium and urea, and also for water absorption. It is also important for the reabsorption of glucose, amino acids, phosphate, calcium and bicarbonate, and for the secretion of H^+.

Glucose

In normal healthy people, almost all of the filtered glucose is reabsorbed and a negligible amount is excreted. Since the normal plasma glucose

Figure 4.3: The relationship of glucose filtration, reabsorption and excretion
to the plasma glucose concentration. The graph is for the normal glomerular
filtration rate (125 mℓ/min). Thus if the plasma glucose concentration is 100
mg/100 mℓ, then 125 mg glucose will be filtered per min. Until the plasma
glucose concentration reaches about 200 mg/100 mℓ, all of the filtered glucose
is reabsorbed and none is excreted. At this concentration (points *a* on the graph),
those nephrons with the poorest ability to reabsorb glucose begin to allow the
excretion of glucose. If the plasma glucose concentration rises further, even those
nephrons with the greatest glucose reabsorptive capacity cannot reabsorb more
(points *b* on the graph). Thus the 'splay' of the curves between points *a* and *b*
indicates nephron inhomogeneity. If all the nephrons had identical glucose
reabsorptive capacities relative to their filtration rate the curves would be as
shown by the dashed lines. The tubular transport maximum for glucose, T_m, is
about 380 mg/min, and is reached when plasma glucose concentration approaches
400 mg/100 mℓ.

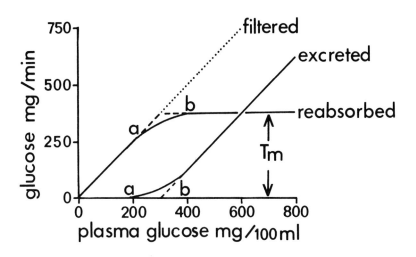

concentration is between 60 and 100 mg/100 mℓ (3.3-5.5 mM) and
the GFR is 125 mℓ/min, it is apparent that between

$$\frac{60 \times 125}{100} = 75 \text{ mg} \quad \text{and} \quad \frac{100 \times 125}{100} = 125 \text{ mg}$$

glucose is reabsorbed every minute.

Although most glucose reabsorption occurs in the proximal tubule,
more distal parts of the nephron are also capable of reabsorbing
glucose. Nevertheless, as the proximal tubule is undoubtedly the major
site of glucose reabsorption, this chapter is the appropriate place to
consider the glucose reabsorptive mechanism. Figure 4.3 shows the

relationship between filtration, reabsorption and excretion of glucose, and the plasma glucose concentration.

The amount of glucose filtered is directly proportional to the plasma glucose concentration. In man, reabsorption of glucose is complete and none is excreted unless the plasma glucose concentration exceeds about 200 mg/100 ml. At this plasma glucose concentration, those nephrons with the lowest capacity for glucose reabsorption (relative to their filtration rate) reach their glucose reabsorptive rate limit, and glucose begins to be excreted. Further increases in plasma glucose concentration saturate the glucose transport process of an increasing proportion of nephrons until, when the plasma glucose concentration is about 400 mg/100 ml, no nephrons are able to absorb all of their filtered glucose load.

If all the nephrons had exactly the same glucose reabsorptive capacity (relative to their filtration rates), we might expect the curves for glucose reabsorption and excretion to be as shown in the dotted lines (Figure 4.3), with a sharp transition from zero excretion to a rate of excretion directly related to the plasma glucose concentration. The fact that the curves are 'splayed' indicates the existence of nephron heterogeneity, i.e. that all the nephrons are not identical.

The type of transport process typified by glucose reabsorption is known as T_m-limited transport. The term T_m means Tubular Maximum, and refers to the maximum tubular reabsorptive capacity for a particular solute. From Figure 4.3 we can see that the maximum rate of glucose reabsorption is about 380 mg/min. This is the T_m for glucose.

Renal abnormalities of glucose excretion, leading to glycosuria, may occur either as a result of a reduced T_m for glucose, or because there is an abnormally wide range of nephron inhomogeneity (i.e. the 'splay' of the glucose excretion curve is increased). Renal glycosuria may occur transiently during pregnancy.

A more serious abnormality of glucose excretion is that caused by a change in the plasma glucose concentration, so that the filtered load is altered: *diabetes mellitus* is caused by the relative or total absence of the pancreatic hormone, insulin, which regulates the blood glucose concentration. In the absence of insulin, the plasma glucose concentration increases, and can exceed 600 mg/100 ml plasma (33 mmol/l). The filtered load of glucose can therefore be far in excess of the reabsorptive capacity of the nephrons, so that glucose is excreted in the urine. This excretion of osmotically active solute causes an osmotic diuresis (see p. 168), resulting in water loss from the body and hence dehydration and thirst.

The Relationship of Glucose Reabsorption to Sodium Reabsorption.
There is considerable evidence indicating that proximal tubular glucose
absorption is indirectly linked to sodium reabsorption, and that there is
a co-transport process for the entry of glucose into the tubular cells
from the lumen, whereby the passive entry of sodium into the cell
down its electrochemical gradient permits the entry of glucose *against*
its gradient. Thus glucose absorption is ultimately dependent on the
maintenance of a gradient for the passive entry of sodium, which in
turn depends on the extrusion of sodium from the peritubular side of
the proximal tubule cells by the sodium pump (Figure 4.4).

Figure 4.4: Co-transport of solutes with sodium. There is evidence that the
reabsorption of a number of substances (e.g. glucose, amino acids, phosphate)
is dependent on sodium reabsorption. Active Na^+ extrusion from the peritubular
side of the proximal tubule cell generates a concentration (and electrical) gradient
for Na^+ entry into the cell from the lumen. Although the Na^+ entry is passive, it
is necessary for Na^+ to be entering the cell in order for molecule X (glucose,
amino acids, phosphate) to enter. The precise molecular nature of this coupling
is unknown.

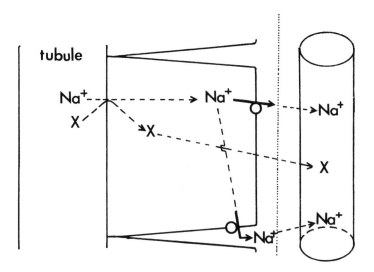

Amino Acids

The plasma concentration of amino acids is 2.5-3.5 mmol/ℓ. Amino acids in the plasma are in a dynamic equilibrium, since they enter the blood from the gut (as products of protein digestion) and are continually being used to restructure the body tissues.

Amino acids are small molecules and are readily filtered at the glomeruli. Negligible quantities of amino acids are excreted, however, because there are effective T_m-limited transport processes for amino acids in the proximal tubule. In fact, there are at least five independent proximal transport processes for amino-acid reabsorption. These are:

(1) for basic amino acids and cystine;
(2) for glutamic and aspartic acids;
(3) for the neutral amino acids;
(4) for imino acids;
(5) for glycine.

The functional characteristics of these transport processes are very similar to that for glucose. Amino-acid entry into the proximal tubule cells from the lumen is a co-transport process with sodium, the driving force being the sodium gradient (Figure 4.4).

Phosphate

Phosphate is an essential constituent of the body. Bones and teeth are salts of calcium and phosphate, and the skeleton accounts for about 80 per cent of the body phosphate content. The other 20 per cent is present mainly in intracellular fluid. The extracellular (plasma) phosphate concentration is 1 mmol/litre (normally expressed as elemental phosphorus — see Chapter 11), and plasma phosphate is freely filtered at the glomerulus. In the nephron, tubular reabsorption and (possibly) secretion of phosphate occurs.

Normally, the urinary phosphate excretion is less than 20 per cent of the amount filtered, but above a phosphate concentration of about 1.2 mmol/ℓ the increments in urinary excretion match the increments in filtration (Figure 4.5), suggesting that there is a T_m for phosphate. Micropuncture studies indicate that this T_m-limited reabsorption occurs in the proximal tubule, but the evidence remains somewhat controversial.

Phosphate reabsorption occurs only in the presence of sodium reabsorption, suggesting a co-transport mechanism. There is evidence that this co-transport occurs in the brush-border membrane but not the

Figure 4.5: The relationship between the plasma phosphate concentration and the amount of phosphate filtered, reabsorbed and excreted. Although superficially similar to the curves for glucose (Figure 4.3), there is an important difference. Whereas the normal amount of glucose filtered is well below the T_m for glucose, the normal amount of phosphate filtered (which of course depends on the plasma concentration) is very close to the T_m for phosphate. Thus the reabsorption process in effect regulates the plasma phosphate concentration, since any increase in plasma phosphate concentration increases phosphate excretion.

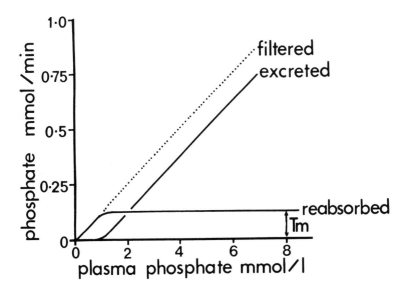

basolateral membrane. The rate of phosphate uptake is hormonally regulated, being under the control of PTH (parathyroid hormone), and vitamin D (Chapter 11).

Urea

The normal plasma urea concentration is 15-45 mg/100 mℓ (2.5-7.5 mmol/ℓ). Whereas virtually 100 per cent of filtered glucose is reabsorbed by the end of the nephron (mainly in the proximal tubule), only 40-50 per cent of filtered urea is reabsorbed and 50-60 per cent is excreted.

Urea is the end product of protein metabolism, and clinically is measured as Blood Urea Nitrogen (BUN). Because urea is a small, lipid-soluble molecule, it is reabsorbed in the proximal tubule as a consequence of sodium reabsorption. Thus, as sodium chloride and water are abstracted from the proximal tubule, the urea concentration in the tubular fluid tends to increase, and so urea is reabsorbed passively by diffusing down its concentration gradient, out of the tubule.

The urea handling of the more distal parts of the nephron plays an important part in the process of concentrating the urine, and is considered later (Chapter 5).

Bicarbonate

The plasma HCO_3^- concentration is normally about 25 mmol/ℓ. Bicarbonate is of great importance in the body because of its key role in acid-base balance, and the kidney contributes to acid-base balance largely by regulating the plasma bicarbonate concentration. How this regulation is accomplished is covered in detail in Chapter 9; at this stage we will consider the basic principles of renal bicarbonate handling.

Figure 4.6: Bicarbonate reabsorption in the proximal tubule. Bicarbonate is filtered into the tubule (left of diagram) at the glomerulus; Na^+ is reabsorbed and H^+ is actively secreted into the tubular lumen. The secreted H^+ combines with HCO_3^- to form carbonic acid (H_2CO_3), which forms CO_2 and H_2O. The formation of CO_2 and H_2O is catalysed by the enzyme carbonic anhydrase, present in the brush border of the proximal tubule cells. Both CO_2 and H_2O can readily enter the tubule cells, where carbonic acid is again formed (catalysed by carbonic anhydrase) and dissociates into H^+ and HCO_3^-. The H^+ is secreted, and HCO_3^- enters the blood together with reabsorbed Na^+ (right of diagram). The end result is that filtered $NaHCO_3$ is reabsorbed and H^+ recycles between cell and tubular lumen.

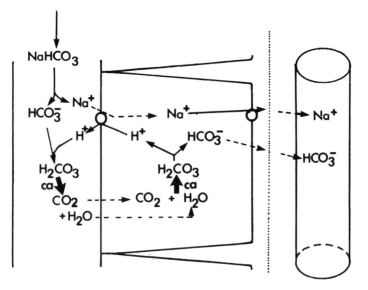

Figure 4.7: The relationship between the plasma bicarbonate concentration and the amount of bicarbonate filtered, reabsorbed and excreted (at a GFR of 125 mℓ/min). The T_m for bicarbonate is variable (as shown by dashed lines), so that the amount excreted at a given plasma concentration also varies (although for clarity the variability in the amount excreted is not shown).

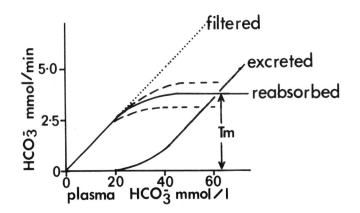

About 90 per cent of the filtered HCO_3^- is reabsorbed in the proximal tubule; the remainder is reabsorbed in the distal tubule and collecting ducts. In the proximal tubule the reabsorption occurs as a result of the active secretion of H^+ from the cells into the tubular lumen. The reaction sequence involved is shown in Figure 4.6.

The bicarbonate reabsorption mechanism behaves *as if* there were a T_m for bicarbonate (Figure 4.7). However, the apparent T_m can be altered by the rate of H^+ secretion, which is itself loosely determined by the rate of Na^+ reabsorption.

Sulphate

Sulphate is reabsorbed in the proximal tubule by an active T_m-limited transport process which serves to maintain the plasma sulphate concentration at 1-1.5 mmol/ℓ.

Secretory Processes in the Proximal Tubule

Tubular secretory mechanisms are very much like tubular reabsorptive mechanisms — the important difference being the direction of transport. Secretion is movement from the peritubular cells into the tubule, whereas reabsorption is movement from the tubule to the cells (and thence to the peritubular fluid). Like reabsorptive processes, secretion can be either active or passive — and active secretory processes may be gradient-time limited (e.g. the proximal tubular hydrogen secretion), or T_m-limited.

There are three proximal tubular secretory mechanisms which have a definite T_m limit, and all three are somewhat puzzling, since most of the T_m-secreted substances do not occur naturally in the body. The three T_m-limited secretory processes are for:

(1) a group of organic acids: these include penicillin, chlorothiazide, hippurate, para-aminohippurate (PAH) and possibly uric acid;
(2) a group of strong organic bases, which includes histamine, choline, thiamine, guanidine and probably creatinine and tetraethylammonium;
(3) EDTA (ethylene diamine tetracetic acid).

Figure 4.8: The filtration, secretion and excretion of PAH, as a function of the plasma PAH concentration. For further explanation see Figure 6.2.

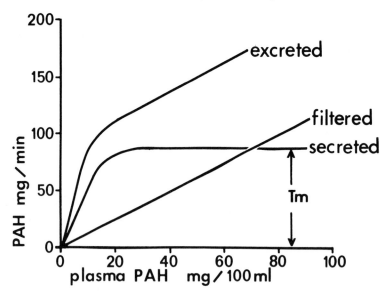

There is some anatomical separation of the different secretory processes. Organic acid secretion (and uric acid secretion) takes place in the pars recta, but organic base secretion occurs in the pars convoluta. It is at present not clear whether these secretion processes are directly coupled to energy consumption, or whether they are co-transport processes with sodium.

PAH, for the physiologist, is a very useful substance, since it can be used to determine renal plasma flow (Chapter 6). Figure 4.8 shows the relationship between the plasma concentration of PAH and the rates of filtration, tubular secretion and urinary excretion.

Over the range of plasma concentrations from 0-8 mg/100 mℓ, PAH secretion can completely remove PAH from the tubular capillaries (thus the only PAH which appears in the renal venous blood is derived from blood which did not go past the proximal tubules). The T_m for the PAH secretory process occurs at a plasma concentration of 10-20 mg/100 mℓ plasma. For further explanation, see Chapter 6, Figure 6.2.

Hydrogen Secretion

In the proximal tubule, H^+ secretion, loosely linked to Na^+ reabsorption, is important in the reabsorption of HCO_3^-. The process is considered in detail in Chapter 9.

Suggestions for Further Reading

Bichara, M., M. Paillard, F. Leviel and J.-P. Gardin. 'Hydrogen transport in rabbit kidney proximal tubules – Na:H exchange', *Am. J. Physiol.*, *238* (1980), pp. F445-51

Giebisch, G. and B. Stanton. 'Potassium transport in the nephron', *Ann. Rev. Physiol.*, *41* (1979), pp. 241-56

Kinne, R. 'Membrane-molecular aspects of tubular transport' in K. Thurau (ed.), *Kidney and Urinary Tract Physiology II*, International Review of Physiology, vol. 11 (University Park Press, Baltimore, 1976), pp. 169-210

Schnermann, J. 'Physical forces and transtubular movement of solutes and water' in K. Thurau (ed.), *Kidney and Urinary Tract Physiology*, MTP International Review of Science, Physiology Series 1, vol. 6 (Butterworths, London, 1974), pp. 157-98

Ullrich, K.J. 'Sugar, amino acid, and Na^+ cotransport in the proximal tubule', *Ann. Rev. Physiol.*, *41* (1979), pp. 181-95

Windhager, E.E. and G. Giebisch. 'Proximal sodium and fluid transport', *Kidney Int.*, *9* (1976), pp. 121-33

5 THE LOOP OF HENLE, DISTAL TUBULE AND COLLECTING DUCT

The Loop of Henle

The fluid entering the loop of Henle is isotonic to plasma, but, after traversing the loop, fluid entering the distal tubule is hypotonic to plasma, i.e. the tubular fluid has been diluted during its passage around the loop of Henle. The length of the loop is related to the maximum possible urinary osmolality; animals with the longest loops of Henle (relative to their kidney size) can produce the most concentrated urine. Only mammals and birds are able to produce concentrated urine (i.e. urine hypertonic to plasma), and only mammals and birds have loops of Henle.

This paradoxical situation — that a nephron segment which dilutes the tubular fluid determines the maximum possible urinary osmolality — was a puzzle to renal physiologists for many years. The solution to the paradox came with the realisation that the loops of Henle are *countercurrent multipliers*, the function of which is not to concentrate the tubular fluid within them, but to manufacture a hypertonic interstitial fluid in the renal medulla. Urine is then concentrated by the osmotic abstraction of water from the collecting ducts as they pass through the medulla.

The Countercurrent Multiplication Mechanism

The theory for the mechanism of countercurrent multiplication in the loop of Henle was propounded by Wirz, Hargitay and Kuhn (1951). Essentially, the theory proposed that if the loop of Henle was able to produce a small osmotic pressure difference between the ascending and descending limbs of the loop (i.e. a small *transverse* gradient), then this small difference would be multiplied into a large *longitudinal gradient* by the countercurrent arrangement (i.e. flow in opposite directions) in the two limbs of the loop.

This theory is now known to be essentially correct. The ascending limb of the loop actively extrudes NaCl into the medullary interstitium, but is impermeable to water, so that water is unable osmotically to follow the ions (Figure 5.1). Consequently, the osmolality of the medullary interstitium is increased, and the osmolality of the fluid in the ascending limb is decreased.

66

Figure 5.1: The fundamental transport processes in the loop of Henle, responsible for the establishment and maintenance of the hypertonicity of the medullary interstitium. NaCl is actively extruded from the ascending limb of Henle's loop. (The process is shown as Cl⁻ active transport, with Na⁺ following, but this is somewhat controversial − see text.) This segment of the nephron is impermeable to H_2O, and the osmolality of the fluid in the ascending limb therefore falls and that of the medullary interstitium increases. The descending limb of Henle's loop is permeable to both ions and water and so comes into osmotic equilibrium with the medullary interstitium. This occurs partly by the movement of NaCl from interstitium to descending limb and party by movement of H_2O from descending limb to interstitium. The transition from water permeability to water impermeability of the tubule is thought to occur at the tip of the loop of Henle. The figures in the diagram show osmolality, mosmoles/kg H_2O.

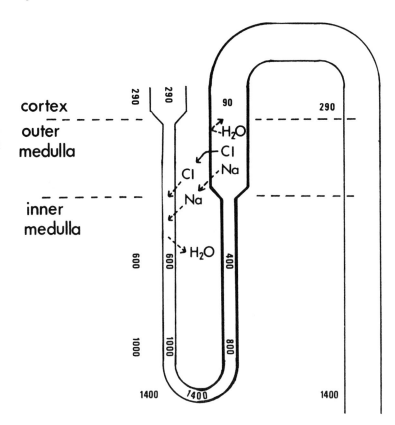

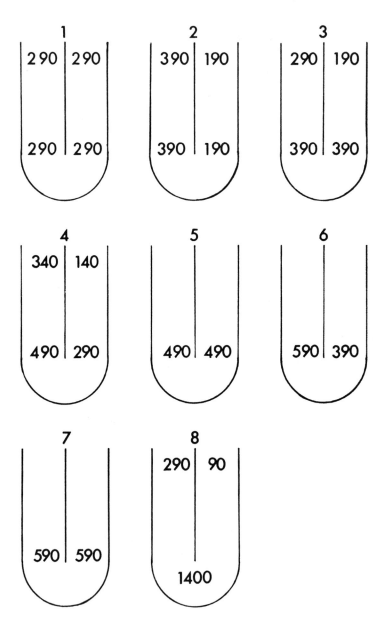

Figure 5.2: Sequence of events in the establishment of the medullary hypertonicity by countercurrent multiplication. It is assumed that the ascending limb of the loop of Henle can produce an osmotic difference of 200 mosmoles/kg H_2O between the tubular lumen and the medullary interstitium. The descending limb attains the same osmolality as the medullary interstitium, and we can therefore regard the transport out of the ascending limb as being directed into the descending limb. In each diagram, the descending limb is on the left and the ascending limb is on the right.

1. Assume that we can start by having the loop of Henle transport processes 'switched off', so that we can fill up the loop with fluid of osmolality 290 mosmoles/kg H_2O from the proximal tubule.

2. If we now operate the NaCl pump in the ascending limb, the pump produces an osmotic difference of 200 mosmoles/kg at each transverse level in the medulla, i.e. the osmolality of the fluid in the ascending limb falls by 100 mosmoles/kg H_2O, and the osmolality of the fluid in the descending limb rises by 100 mosmoles/kg H_2O.

3. We now move the contents of the loop round, ejecting fluid into the distal tubule and introducing more fluid of osmolality 290 from the proximal tubule.

4. Operation of the NaCl pump again to maintain a difference of 200 mosmoles/kg H_2O between ascending and descending limbs.

5. Ejection of more fluid into distal tubule, and introduction into descending limb of fluid with osmolality 290 from proximal tubule. Fluid at the tip of the loop is moved round so that fluid of osmolality 490 is present at bottom of ascending and descending limbs. For simplicity, only the osmolalities at the tip of the loop are shown.

6. Operation of NaCl pump.

7. Further flow around loop so that fluid of osmolality 590 is present at bottom of both limbs.

8. Gradient fully established. Fluid entering descending limb from proximal tubule has an osmolality of 290 mosmoles/kg H_2O. Fluid leaving the ascending limb into the distal tubule has an osmolality of about 90 mosmoles/kg H_2O. The osmolality at the tip of the loop is 1,400, but the difference in osmolalities between ascending and descending limbs at any transverse level is only 200 mosmoles/kg H_2O. The interstitial osmolality is the same as that of the descending limb.

Whether it is Cl^- or Na^+ which is actively transported out of the ascending limb of the loop of Henle remains uncertain. (There is considerable evidence that Cl^- is actively transported, but a recent study (Greger, 1981) indicates that the process is Na-Cl co-transport, such that Cl^- entry into the cells from the lumen is a sodium-dependent process, driven by the Na^+-K^+-ATPase which extrudes Na^+ across the basolateral membrane.) The ascending limb is impermeable to water, so that water is unable osmotically to follow the ions. Consequently, the osmolality of the medullary interstitium is increased and the osmolality of the fluid in the ascending limb is decreased.

To examine the process of countercurrent multiplication in detail, let us imagine that we can 'turn off' the active processes which occur in the loop of Henle, and then fill up the loop with isotonic fluid (osmolality 290 mosmoles/kg H_2O) from the proximal tubule (refer to Figure 5.2).

The cells in the wall of the ascending limb are able to sustain an osmotic pressure difference between the luminal side and interstitial side (i.e. a transverse gradient) of about 200 mosmoles/kg H_2O. So if the fluid in the ascending limb in our hypothetical situation (before we turn on the pump) has an osmolality of 290 mosmoles/kg H_2O, the pump can lower the luminal osmolality to 190 mosmoles/kg and raise the interstitial osmolality to 390 mosmoles/kg. This sequence of events is shown in Figure 5.2.

The descending limb is permeable to water, and to a lesser extent is also permeable to NaCl. The fluid within the descending limb will therefore come to osmotic equilibrium with the interstitium. In effect, then, we can consider the transport of NaCl out of the ascending limb as being directed into the descending limb.

With the above, we are now in possession of all the facts necessary to understand how the countercurrent multiplication system works, and in Figure 5.2 the process is artificially divided into a series of separate stages. In stage 1, the loop is filled up with isotonic fluid from the proximal tubule. In stage 2, we operate the NaCl pump in the ascending limb, which produces a 200 mosmole/kg H_2O gradient between the ascending and the descending limb. If we now (stage 3) move more isotonic fluid in from the proximal tubule, and move some of the hypertonic fluid around the bend from the descending to the ascending limb, we can establish a new equilibrium (stage 4) by operation of the NaCl pump. As this sequence continues (stages 5 to 8), the osmolality at the tip of the loop (and in the interstitium) progressively increases. In man, the osmolality at the papilla tip can reach 1,400 mosmoles/kg H_2O, i.e. about five times the plasma osmolality. So, with the countercurrent multiplier, the small transverse gradient (200 mosmoles/kg H_2O) can be converted into a considerable longitudinal gradient.

So far, a number of details have been omitted from this scheme. The structure of the ascending limb of the loop of Henle is not uniform, there being a thin segment and a thick segment (Figure 5.1). Both segments are impermeable to water, but it may be that only the thick segment actively extrudes NaCl. However, this does not affect the basic principle of the countercurrent arrangement, which still depends on the removal of NaCl from the ascending limb, unaccompanied by water.

As a result of the countercurrent multiplication mechanism, the fluid in the tubules leaving the medulla and entering the cortex is hypotonic to plasma, with an osmolality of about 100 mosmoles/kg H_2O. Thus the ascending limb of the loop of Henle (and its continuation in the cortex as the anatomically defined 'distal tubule') can be called the 'diluting segment' of the nephron.

The fact that the 'distal tubule' is not a distinct section of the nephron physiologically is responsible for the considerable confusion concerning the functions of this segment. The problem arises from the fact that different species, different strains of animals, and even different individuals, vary in the point at which ascending-limb-of-Henle-type cells are replaced by collecting-tubule-type cells. The walls of the former cell type have only a low (and essentially constant) permeability to water whereas the walls of the collecting-duct-type cells have a variable water permeability, regulated by the hormone ADH (antidiuretic hormone, vasopressin).

The potential difference across the distal tubular region varies with distance along the tubule. In the early part, the lumen is positive (as in the ascending limb of Henle), but in the later parts the luminal potential (relative to plasma) is negative and may reach −45 mV. This negative potential is caused by active sodium reabsorption.

The Collecting Tubules

The collecting tubules have cortical and medullary sections and the two sections have somewhat different properties.

The cortical and medullary sections are both relatively impermeable to water, urea and NaCl, but the *water permeability is increased by ADH*. Thus ADH leads to urine concentration by permitting the osmotic abstraction of water into the interstitium, so that the urine in the collecting tubule can theoretically achieve the same osmolality (up to 1,400 mosmoles/kg H_2O) as the medullary interstitium, although it is usually rather less than this. Water reabsorbed from the medullary collecting tubules will tend to dilute the medullary interstitium, so that, for the concentration process to remain effective, the fluid delivery to the medullary collecting tubule (i.e. the fluid available for reabsorption in the medulla) must be small in volume. This is brought about (under the influence of ADH) by water reabsorption in the cortical collecting tubules. It was mentioned above that the osmolality of the fluid leaving the distal tubule is about 100 mosmoles/ kg H_2O. (This is normally not more than 15 per cent of the glomerular filtrate, the rest having already been absorbed in the proximal tubule and loop of Henle.) In the presence of ADH, water reabsorption in the cortical collecting tubule will account for about 66 per cent of the fluid delivered to it (i.e. it will be concentrated from 100 to 290 mosmoles/ kg by osmotic abstraction of water) leaving less than 5 per cent of the glomerular filtrate to continue into the medullary collecting tubules.

ADH increases the *urea permeability* of the medullary collecting tubules, but has no effect on the urea permeability of the cortical collecting tubules. This impermeability of the cortical part of the collecting tubule is one of the factors which makes urea so important in the urine concentration mechanism.

Importance of Urea in Countercurrent Multiplication

Although we have so far considered the countercurrent multiplication process only in terms of NaCl transport into the interstitium, a considerable fraction of the interstitial osmotic pressure is attributable to urea. The normal plasma concentration of urea is 15-45 mg/100 mℓ (i.e. 2.5-7.5 mmol/ℓ). Urea is freely filterable at the glomerulus, and approximately 50 per cent of the filtered load is reabsorbed (passively) in the proximal tubule. As the tubular fluid passes down the descending limb of the loop of Henle, the urea concentration *increases*, as a result of the diffusion of urea from the interstitium, down a concentration gradient, into the tubule (why there is such a high urea concentration in the medullary interstitium will soon be apparent).

When the tubular fluid reaches the 'distal tubule' and cortical collecting tubule, the urea concentration rises still more, as a result of water reabsorption, since these segments are almost impermeable to urea. When the medullary collecting tubule is reached, the high urea concentration in the tubule causes the diffusion of urea out of the tubule into the interstitium (the medullary collecting tubule is permeable to urea in the presence of ADH) thereby raising the interstitial urea concentration and so causing diffusion of urea into the descending limb of the loop of Henle. Thus urea recycles in the medulla, as shown in Figure 5.3.

Since the papillary osmolality is due in part (up to 50 per cent) to urea, the papillary osmolality is increased by increasing ADH levels, because in the presence of ADH the medullary collecting tubule is

Figure 5.3: Trapping of urea in the medullary interstitium. Urea is delivered to the loop of Henle from the proximal tubule, and passes round the loop of Henle to enter the distal tubule and thence the collecting ducts. In the presence of ADH water is reabsorbed from the cortical collecting ducts, but this segment is impermeable to urea, and therefore the luminal urea concentration increases. In the medullary collecting ducts, in the presence of ADH, both urea and water can leave the tubule, and urea diffuses down its concentration gradient into the medullary interstitium. The high interstitial urea concentration thus achieved leads to the diffusion of some urea into the loop of Henle, to return to the collecting duct.

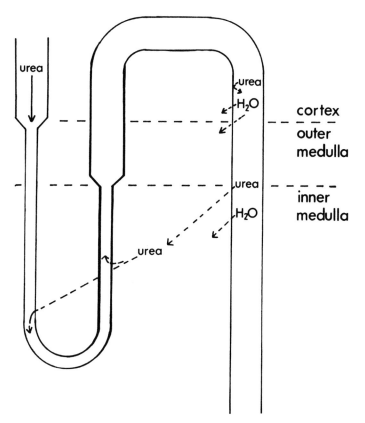

permeable to urea so that urea diffuses into the interstitium. Also, the maximum attainable urinary osmolality is greater when urea excretion is high than when urea excretion is low (urea is a product of protein metabolism, so a high protein diet increases urea excretion), because a proportion of this extra urea enters the medullary interstitium.

Further Requirements of the Countercurrent Multiplication Mechanism: The Vasa Recta

The vasa recta are capillaries, mostly derived from the efferent arterioles of juxtamedullary nephrons, which have a 'hairpin' arrangement and dip far down into the renal medulla.

Figure 5.4: Countercurrent exchange in the vasa recta. (a) As the descending vasa recta enter the increasingly hypertonic medullary interstitium, water is osmotically abstracted from the blood vessel, so that the osmolality of the blood (and its viscosity) are increased. In the ascending limb, water re-enters the blood vessel. The system ensures a low flow rate through the deep parts of the vasa recta, and minimises the washout of medullary solutes. (b) O_2 and CO_2 also undergo countercurrent exchange in the vasa recta, so that the vasa recta are rather inefficient suppliers of O_2 and removers of CO_2 for cells deep in the medulla.

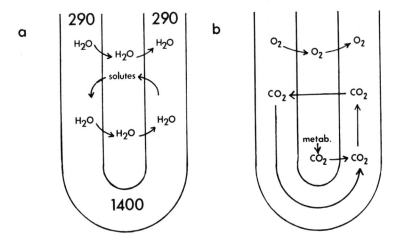

In parts of the body other than the renal medulla, the circulation of blood through capillaries (which are freely permeable to water and small molecules) ensures the uniformity of the composition of the interstitial fluid. If the medullary capillaries served a similar purpose, the osmotic gradient built up by the loop of Henle would be dissipated. This does not occur, because the hairpin arrangement of the vasa recta enables them to function as *countercurrent exchangers* (distinguished from countercurrent multipliers by the fact that no energy is necessary). Thus, the function of the vasa recta is to provide nutrients to, and remove waste products from, the renal medulla, without washing away the solutes responsible for medullary hypertonicity.

The vasa recta, like capillaries elsewhere, are permeable to water and solutes. So, as plasma in the descending vasa recta passes down into the medulla, water will be osmotically abstracted from the vasa recta into the interstitium and solutes (NaCl and urea) will enter (Figure 5.4). More and more water will come out as the blood passes further into the medulla, until, at the tip of the loop, the plasma has almost the same osmolality as the surrounding interstitium and the blood is very viscous (with a high plasma protein concentration as a result of water loss to the interstitium). In the ascending vasa recta, the plasma regains the water and loses most of the solutes.

Some solutes are, however, washed out from the medulla, but if this were not the case, there might be no limit to how hypertonic the interstitium could become (i.e. theoretically countercurrent multiplication could go on *ad infinitum*). Other limiting factors for the degree of hypertonicity attained in the interstitium are the volumes of water reabsorbed from the collecting ducts and descending loops of Henle (most of this water enters the vasa recta and is removed from the medulla), and diffusion of solutes longitudinally within the medullary interstitium.

Long and Short Loops of Henle

It has been mentioned (Chapter 2) that, in man, only 15 per cent of the nephrons (the juxtamedullary nephrons) have long loops of Henle which pass deeply into the medulla. The remaining 85 per cent of nephrons (cortical nephrons) have short loops of Henle which barely reach the medulla.

The nephrons with short loops of Henle do not make a significant contribution to the manufacture of medullary hypertonicity. However, the collecting tubules of *all* the nephrons (both cortical and juxtamedullary), pass through the medulla; thus, the long-looped nephrons, which are 15 per cent of the total, produce a medullary gradient which leads to the concentration of urine from all the nephrons.

The Regulation of Urine Concentration

The urine osmolality can range from about 60 mosmoles/kg H_2O up to 1,400 mosmoles/kg H_2O, and the volume per 24 hours can be as little as 300 mℓ or as much as 23 litres. How are such dramatic changes brought about?

The main determinant of whether the urine will be copious and dilute, or small in volume and concentrated, is the level of circulating ADH (antidiuretic hormone, vasopressin). The ways in which the level of ADH is regulated are considered later (Chapters 7 and 8). At this stage, we will simply look at the effects of altering the level of circulating ADH. This section will also serve to summarise the information we have covered so far concerning urine production.

Maximal ADH. The Production of Concentrated Urine (Figure 5.5)

The reabsorption of water in the nephron occurs at several sites. The glomerular filtration rate is 180 ℓ/day, and approximately 70 per cent of this is reabsorbed in the proximal tubule, so that about 53 ℓ/day of *isotonic* fluid is delivered to the loops of Henle.

A further 5 per cent (approximately 10 ℓ/day) of the glomerular filtrate is reabsorbed by the (descending limb of the) loop of Henle, leaving 43 ℓ/day to enter the 'distal tubule'. The 'distal tubule' reabsorbs approximately 10 per cent of the filtered load (about 20 ℓ/day), leaving 23 litres to enter the collecting tubules. It is this 23 litres which can be either mainly excreted or mainly reabsorbed depending on the level of circulating ADH. In the presence of ADH the collecting tubule wall is permeable to water, so water reabsorption occurs. Cortical absorption accounts for 66 per cent of the water entering the collecting tubules (in the presence of ADH; see section above on collecting tubules), so the delivery of fluid to the medullary collecting tubule is low (8 ℓ/day approximately), and as this fluid passes down the tubule, the hypertonic medullary interstitium leads to the osmotic abstraction of water from the tubule. Urea also leaves the tubule in this region. The urine volume in these circumstances can be as little as 300 mℓ/day.

No circulating ADH. The Production of Dilute Urine (Figure 5.6)

In the absence of circulating ADH, water reabsorption in the proximal and distal tubules occurs as above — i.e. ADH does not affect water absorption at these sites. However, the impermeability of the collecting tubules in the absence of ADH means that a large volume of water enters the medullary collecting tubule and is excreted. In addition, the impermeability of medullary collecting tubules to urea prevents the attainment of maximal medullary interstitial tonicity, and this in turn may slightly reduce water reabsorption from the descending limb of the loop of Henle. So ADH not only determines the urine volume,

Figure 5.5: Water reabsorption in the collecting duct in the presence of maximal plasma levels of ADH. The figures show tubular fluid osmolality. Abbreviations: p.t., proximal tubule; l.h., loop of Henle; d.t., distal tubule; c.c.d., cortical collecting duct; m.c.d., medullary collecting duct. In the proximal tubule, water and solute reabsorption occur, but the tubular fluid remains isotonic to plasma (osmolality 290 mosmoles/kg H_2O). In the loop of Henle, countercurrent multiplication produces an osmolality at the tip of the loop, of 1,400 mosmoles/kg H_2O. Fluid entering the distal tubule is hypotonic. Some water is absorbed in the distal tubule, but sodium chloride reabsorption also occurs and the tubular fluid remains hypotonic (90 mosmoles/kg H_2O). In the cortical collecting duct, water absorption occurs in the presence of ADH and the tubular fluid becomes isotonic to plasma (290 mosmoles/kg H_2O); the volume of fluid delivered to the medullary collecting duct is small and water absorption along the osmotic gradient into the medullary interstitium raises the tubular fluid osmolality to close to 1,400 mosmoles/kg H_2O. Note that some sodium absorption occurs in the collecting ducts.

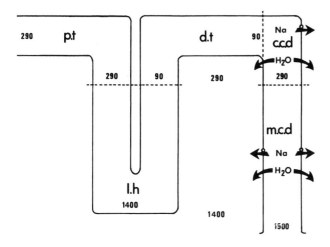

but also influences the medullary tonicity.

Normally, there is some ADH present in the circulation, and the urine volume is approximately 1.5 ℓ/day, with an osmolality of 300-500 mosmoles/kg H_2O, but in the absence of ADH urine volume is approximately 23 ℓ/day, with an osmolality as low as 60 mosmoles/kg H_2O (diabetes insipidus).

It should be noted that adrenal steroids (cortisol) must be present if very dilute urine is to be produced.

Figure 5.6: Water reabsorption in the collecting duct in the absence of ADH. For abbreviations, see Figure 5.5. Events in the proximal tubule are identical to those in Figure 5.5. In the loop of Henle, the tubular fluid becomes hypertonic, but the gradient is lower than in the presence of ADH (see text). Distal tubular events are as in Figure 5.5. In the cortical collecting duct, in the absence of ADH, water reabsorption does not occur. Sodium reabsorption therefore tends to lower the tubular fluid osmolality still further. This process continues in the medullary collecting duct and a large volume of very dilute urine is produced.

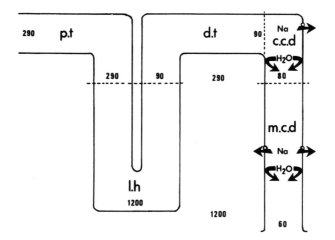

Suggestions for Further Reading

Berl, T., G.L. Robertson, G.A. Aisenbury, R.W. Schrier and R.J. Anderson. 'Role of vasopressin in the impaired water excretion of glucocorticoid deficiency', *Kidney Int., 18* (1980), pp. 58-67

Berliner, R.W. 'The concentrating mechanism in the renal medulla', *Kidney Int., 9* (1976), pp. 214-22

Greger, R. 'Chloride reabsorption in the rabbit cortical thick ascending limb of Henle's loop of rabbit kidney', *Pflügers Arch., 390* (1981), pp. 38-43

Jamison, R.L. and C.R. Robertson. 'Recent formulations of the urinary concentrating mechanism: a status report', *Kidney Int., 16* (1979), pp. 537-45

Rector, F.C. Jr. 'Renal concentrating mechanisms' in T.E. Andreoli, J.J. Grantham and F.C. Rector Jr (eds), *Disturbances in Body Fluid Osmolality* (American Physiological Society, Washington, 1977), pp. 179-96

Schwarz, M.J. and J.P. Kokko. 'Urinary concentrating defect in adrenal insufficiency', *J. Clin. Invest., 66* (1980), pp. 234-42

Wirz, H., B. Hargitay and W. Kuhn. 'Lokalisation des konzentrierungs-prozesses in der niere durch direkte kryoskopie', *Helv. Physiol. Pharmacol. Acta, 9* (1951), pp. 196-207

6 RENAL BLOOD FLOW AND GLOMERULAR FILTRATION RATE

Since the functioning of the kidneys depends on filtration of the plasma, the blood flow to the kidneys is of obvious importance. How the blood flow and glomerular filtration rate are regulated is the subject of the second part of this chapter. First, the measurement of renal blood flow (RBF) and glomerular filtration rate (GFR) will be considered.

Measurement of Renal Blood Flow and Glomerular Filtration Rate

In order to discuss the ways in which renal blood flow and glomerular filtration rate can be measured, the concept of *clearance* must be introduced. The clearance of any substance excreted by the kidney is the *volume of plasma* which is cleared of the substance in unit time. The units of clearance are volume/time, usually $m\ell/min$.

Consider the clearance of a substance, x. Clearance is given by the formula

$$C_x = \frac{U_x V}{P_x}$$

where C_x is the clearance of x, U_x is the urine conc. of substance x, P_x is the plasma conc. of substance x and V is the urine flow ($m\ell/min$). If we express the formula in terms of the units of measurement

$$C_x = \frac{U_x \text{ mg}/m\ell \cdot V \, m\ell/min}{P_x \text{ mg}/m\ell}$$

it should be obvious that the units of clearance are $m\ell/min$.

In fact, the clearance represents a *theoretical* volume of plasma which is completely cleared of the substance, x, in 1 min, because in reality, no aliquot of plasma is *completely* cleared of any substance by its passage through the kidney. Nevertheless, the clearance formula has considerable usefulness in renal physiology and for assessing renal function in disease. Below, we consider the clearances of two specific substances, inulin and *p*-aminohippuric acid, which can be used to measure the glomerular filtration rate and the renal plasma flow, respectively.

Before we look at the clearance of these substances in detail, an understanding of the technical requirements for accurate clearance measurements is necessary. Because the plasma concentration of the substance, x, must be known accurately, it must be either constant or changing in a predictable way so that an accurate average concentration can be calculated. So clearance measurements are only suitable for the steady-state determinations of GFR and RBF, and cannot be used if rapid or transient changes are occurring. An additional complication is that urine flow must be adequate to collect sufficient for the assay in the clearance period (which is usually 10-20 min), so clearance measurements are not possible in conditions of anuria.

Inulin Clearance: The Measurement of Glomerular Filtration Rate

Inulin is a polysaccharide with a molecular weight of approximately 5,500. It is not a normal constituent of the body, but can be injected (or, usually, infused) intravenously in order to measure the inulin clearance.

Inulin is small enough to pass through the glomerular filter without difficulty, but is neither reabsorbed, secreted, synthesised nor metabolised by the kidney. So all of the filtered inulin is excreted, and all the inulin which is excreted has entered the urine only by filtration at the glomerulus.

The amount of inulin excreted per minute is $U_{in} V$, i.e. the urinary inulin concentration, U_{in} (mg/mℓ) multiplied by the urine flow, V (mℓ/min) and therefore this is the amount which entered the nephron by being contained in filtered plasma. The volume of plasma from which the amount $U_{in} V$ mg/min of inulin was derived must therefore have been

$$\frac{U_{in} V}{P_{in}} \quad \text{m}\ell/\text{min}$$

and this is the clearance formula, where P_{in} is the plasma concentration of inulin (mg/mℓ).

Thus the inulin clearance, C_{in}, is equal to the glomerular filtration rate (GFR). The inulin clearance measurement (and hence the GFR measurement) is independent of the plasma inulin concentration, as the graph in Figure 6.1 shows.

The normal inulin clearance (GFR) is 125 mℓ/min (180 litres/day; it varies with body size; the value is really 125 mℓ/min/1.73 m^2 body surface area). Even taking into account body surface area, GFR is low

Figure 6.1: Inulin filtered and excreted as a function of plasma concentration. Since, after filtration, inulin is neither reabsorbed nor secreted, the amount excreted is identical to the amount filtered. The amount excreted (mg/min) is calculated as the product of the urinary inulin concentration, U_{in}, and the urine flow, V. The inulin clearance, $U_{in}V/P_{in}$, is independent of the plasma inulin concentration (P_{in}), e.g. if P_{in} is 2 mg/100 mℓ (0.02 mg/mℓ) then $U_{in}V/P_{in}$, from the graph, is 2.5/0.02 = 125 mℓ/min. If P_{in} is 4 mg/100 mℓ (0.04 mg/mℓ) then $U_{in}V/P_{in}$ is 5/0.04 = 125 mℓ/min again.

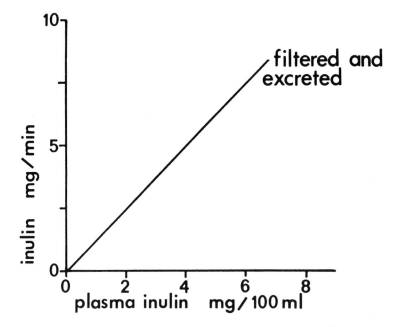

in infants and decreases in old age. From day to day the GFR is remarkably constant in man. Variations in excretion of water and solutes depend on changes in tubular reabsorption and secretion, not on GFR changes.

Because inulin is not a normal constituent of the body, and measurements of inulin clearance therefore involve inulin infusions, it is rarely used clinically. A suitable alternative way to measure GFR is by using *creatinine clearance*. Creatinine is a product of muscle metabolism, so, as long as the subject remains at rest, plasma creatinine level stays reasonably constant. Like inulin, it is freely filtered and not reabsorbed, synthesised or metabolised by the kidney. However, creatinine is secreted to some extent by the tubules, which makes the term *UV* artifactually high, but as the plasma creatinine assay is not absolutely specific and overestimates the true plasma creatinine concentration, the two errors tend to cancel each other and creatinine clearance is a reasonable estimate of GFR.

PAH Clearance: The Measurement of Renal Plasma Flow

PAH (para-aminohippuric acid) is one of the group of organic acids which are actively secreted by the proximal tubule. The secretory process is T_m-limited (see Chapter 4). PAH is not only secreted, but is also filtered at the glomerulus. Thus the amount excreted is equal to the sum of the amount filtered, plus the amount secreted. This is illustrated graphically in Figure 6.2.

Figure 6.2: The relationship between plasma p-aminohippuric acid (PAH) concentration and the filtration, secretion and excretion of PAH (at a GFR of 125 mℓ/min). In addition to being filtered, PAH is also actively secreted, so the amount excreted/min is the sum of the amount filtered/min plus the amount secreted/min. The T_m for PAH secretion is reached at a rather low plasma PAH concentration (approximately 10 mg/100 mℓ).

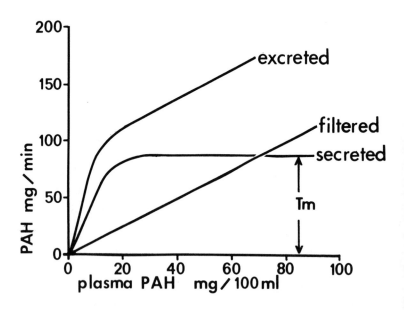

The T_m for PAH is reached at a plasma concentration of about 10 mg/100 mℓ plasma. At plasma concentrations below this, the clearance of PAH provides us with a measurement of the renal plasma flow (RPF). Why is this? In order to understand how PAH clearance can be a measure of RPF, it is necessary to introduce the *Fick* principle. The Fick principle is generally used to measure the lung blood flow — which is the same as the cardiac output. The formula is as follows

lung blood flow (i.e. cardiac output)

$$= \frac{\text{oxygen uptake/min}}{\text{arteriovenous oxygen concentration difference}}$$

Expressed in mathematical terms, this becomes

$$\text{lung blood flow} = \frac{\dot{Q}_{O_2}}{A_{O_2} - V_{O_2}}$$

where $\dot{Q}_{O_2}$ = ml of O_2 used per min, A_{O_2} = arterial O_2 conc., V_{O_2} = venous O_2 conc. (The formula could also be applied using CO_2 output instead of O_2 uptake.)

The formula can be applied to any organ in which the blood takes up or loses any substance. So, in the kidney, let us suppose that the substance 'x' is removed from the blood during its passage through the organ. Then:

$$\text{Renal blood flow} = \frac{\text{Amount 'x' excreted/min}}{\text{Arteriovenous concentration difference of 'x'}}$$

$$= \frac{U_x V}{A_x - V_x}$$

where $U_x V$ is amount of x (mg) excreted per min, A_x is the renal arterial conc. of x, V_x is the renal venous conc. of x.

As long as the T_m is not exceeded, PAH is almost completely removed from the blood, and consequently the renal venous conc. can be considered to be zero. So applying the Fick formula to PAH, we can say

$$\text{Renal blood flow} = \frac{U_{PAH} V}{A_{PAH} - V_{PAH}}$$

but since V_{PAH} is zero,

$$\text{RBF} = \frac{U_{PAH} V}{A_{PAH}}$$

where A_{PAH} is, strictly, the renal arterial conc. of PAH. However, a venous concentration measurement can be used, provided that the venous sample does not include *renal* venous blood. This is usually the case because samples are generally taken from a limb, where the venous concentration is equal to the renal arterial concentration. In fact, since only plasma PAH is filtered, and we normally only measure PAH in the *plasma* (not whole blood), we measure the renal plasma flow (RPF) as

$$\text{Clearance of PAH} = \text{RPF} = \frac{U_{PAH}V}{P_{PAH}}$$

where P_{PAH} is the plasma PAH concentration. A typical figure for RPF obtained in this way is 600 mℓ/min.

We can then use the haematocrit to obtain the renal blood flow, e.g. the usual haematocrit is 45 per cent. This means that 45 per cent of the total blood volume is cells and therefore 55 per cent is plasma. Therefore

$$\text{RBF} = \text{RPF} \times \frac{100}{55}$$

$$= 600 \times \frac{100}{55} \simeq 1100 \text{ m}\ell/\text{min}$$

The clearance of PAH, although generally used as a measure of renal plasma flow, in fact does not measure the plasma flow exactly. This is because PAH is not completely cleared from the blood during one passage through the kidney. The PAH extraction is about 90 per cent complete. This incomplete removal is due to the fact that not all of the blood which enters the kidney goes to the glomeruli and tubules. Some goes to the capsule, the perirenal fat and the medulla (the blood in the vasa recta has had some PAH removed by filtration, but is not available for secretion). The PAH clearance approximates *cortical* plasma flow, and is usually called the Effective Renal Plasma Flow (ERPF).

Filtration Fraction

As inulin clearance is a measure of glomerular filtration rate, and PAH clearance is a measure of the effective renal plasma flow, simultaneous measurements of inulin and PAH clearance enable us to calculate the fraction of renal plasma that is filtered through the glomeruli into the nephrons.

$$\text{Filtration fraction} = \frac{C_{in}}{C_{PAH}} = \frac{125 \text{ m}\ell/\text{min}}{600 \text{ m}\ell/\text{min}} \simeq 20\% \text{ in normal man}$$

Other Ways of Measuring Renal Blood Flow

Clearance methods cannot tell us anything about the distribution of blood flow within the kidney. Several methods are available, however, which can provide information about the distribution of blood flow in experimental animals.

The Inert Gas 'Washout' Technique. This procedure is as follows: a small volume of saline containing radioactive krypton (^{85}Kr), or xenon (^{133}Xe) is administered by rapid injection into a renal artery (via a catheter). The lipid-soluble gas rapidly diffuses across the renal capillary membranes, so that the renal tissue becomes almost instantaneously saturated with the gas. The rate of removal ('washout') of the gas from tissue will then depend on the blood flow.

Isotope Uptake Technique. ^{42}K or ^{86}Rb (radioactive potassium or rubidium) is administered by rapid intravenous injection, and the animal is then killed. The rate of accumulation of the isotope in the different segments of renal tissue provides a measure of the blood flow through the regions.

The Regulation of Renal Blood Flow and Glomerular Filtration Rate

Because the function of the renal blood supply is to provide blood for filtration, it is clear that an adequate supply of blood to the kidney is necessary if the normal excretory functions of the kidney are to continue. We have already seen that the renal blood supply is very large (about 1.1 ℓ/min, or 20 per cent of the cardiac output). An important feature of the renal blood flow is that, over a wide range of perfusion pressures (from a mean of 90 mm Hg up to about 200 mm Hg), the blood flow is independent of the perfusion pressure. This is true even if the kidney is denervated – i.e. it does not depend on the renal nerve supply. It also occurs in isolated perfused kidneys, so does not depend on blood-borne hormones. This property is therefore termed 'autoregulation' (Figure 6.3). The glomerular filtration rate also autoregulates (Figure 6.3). Essentially, the relationship between blood pressure and renal blood flow demonstrated in Figure 6.3 means that as the perfusion pressure increases, the resistance to flow also increases. Both afferent arterioles and efferent arterioles are capable of vasoconstriction. The effects are explained in Figure 6.4.

There is still some controversy about precisely how the autoregulation

Figure 6.3: The autoregulation of glomerular filtration rate (dotted line) and renal blood flow (solid line). In the autoregulatory range (90-200 mm Hg), changes in mean arterial blood pressure (BP) have little effect on the renal blood flow (RBF) or the glomerular filtration rate (GFR).

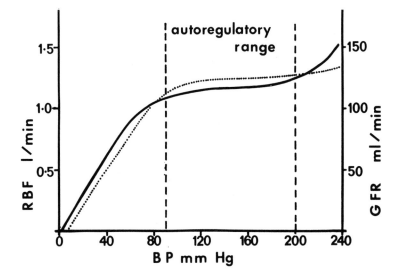

of renal blood flow and GFR occurs. The most widely accepted explanation is the *myogenic theory*, according to which the increase in wall tension of the afferent arterioles, brought about by an increase in perfusion pressure, causes automatic contraction of the smooth muscle fibres in the vessel wall, thereby increasing the resistance to flow and so keeping the flow constant in spite of the increase in perfusion pressure. There is considerable experimental evidence in support of this hypothesis.

Further Points Concerning Renal Haemodynamics

Because the kidneys exhibit the property of autoregulation it is easy to forget that renal haemodynamics do vary considerably. Autoregulation means that changes in blood pressure *per se*, in the autoregulatory range, have little effect on blood flow. It does *not* mean that blood flow is always constant. In many circumstances (e.g. physical or mental stress, haemorrhage), there are increases in the sympathetic nervous activity to the kidney (and to other parts of the body), causing vasoconstriction and hence a reduction in renal blood flow, even though the perfusion pressure is still in the autoregulatory

Figure 6.4: Diagram to show the ways in which vasoconstriction can occur in the afferent arterioles (*aa*) and efferent arterioles (*ea*) on either side of the glomerular capillary bed (*gc*). GFR and RBF are maintained constant by the combination of afferent and efferent arteriolar vasoconstrictor activity. (a) Normal situation, such as would occur at mean arterial blood pressure of 100 mm Hg. (b) Afferent arteriolar constriction in response to an increase of mean arterial blood pressure. The constriction of the afferent arteriole reduces the glomerular capillary pressure below what it would otherwise be, and both GFR and RBF can stay constant in spite of the increased arterial blood pressure. (c) Efferent arteriolar constriction increases the GFR (i.e. a larger fraction of the plasma delivered to the kidney is filtered).

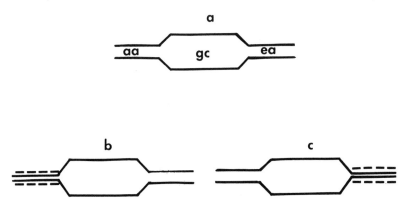

range. But when renal blood flow is reduced, there is generally an increased filtration fraction brought about by efferent arteriolar constriction, so that GFR tends to be maintained.

Suggestions for Further Reading

Barger, A.C. and J.A. Herd. 'Renal vascular anatomy and distribution of blood flow' in J. Orloff and R.W. Berliner (eds), *Handbook of Physiology 8, Renal Physiology* (American Physiological Society, Washington, 1973), pp. 249-313
Stein, J.H. 'The renal circulation' in B.M. Brenner and F.C. Rector (eds), *The Kidney*, vol. 1 (Saunders, Philadelphia, 1976), pp. 215-50

7 THE REGULATION OF BODY FLUID OSMOLALITY

Introduction

The body weight of a healthy adult on an adequate diet remains remarkably stable from day to day, and this stability indicates that the body fluid volume is staying constant, i.e. there is a steady state, in which the fluid output equals the fluid input. The normal intake and output of water over a 24-hour period is shown below.

Intake (ml)		Output (ml)	
Drinking	1500	Urine	1500
Water in food	500	Respiration	400
Metabolism	400	Skin	400
	———	Faeces	100
Total	2400		———
		Total	2400

It can be seen that water is lost from the body via several routes. The loss from the skin is 'insensible perspiration' and it occurs continually. Sweating (or 'sensible' perspiration) represents an additional loss (not shown in the table, but it can be up to 5 ℓ/hr). The loss from the respiratory tract occurs because inspired air is moistened as it passes to the lungs, and some of this moisture is then lost from the body in the expired air. This loss is greater in very dry environments, such as in deserts or in subzero temperatures. The faecal loss is normally small, but in pathological states faecal losses can lead to very severe dehydration — which may frequently be the cause of death, e.g. in cholera. This is because the gastrointestinal tract not only has to reabsorb the water taken in by mouth (1500 mℓ/day), but also must reabsorb the secreted digestive juices (up to 20 ℓ/day). Failure to do so leads to very large water losses. Such losses can be more serious in young infants and serious body fluid disturbances may occur as a result of diarrhoea.

From the foregoing, it is apparent that the fluid losses from the skin and respiratory tract, and in the faeces, are potential disturbing factors for body fluid balance. In contrast, the loss from the kidney can be regulated, so that the loss of fluid in the urine and the urine composition are adjusted to keep the body fluid volume and composition

88

constant. (There are, of course, limits to the regulatory capacity of the kidney. If no water at all is ingested, then the urine becomes maximally concentrated and small in volume, but urinary water loss cannot be reduced below about 300 mℓ/day.)

The normal plasma osmolality (P_{osm}) is 280-290 mosmoles/kg H_2O; it is regulated very precisely, and a variation in either direction of about 3 mosmoles/kg H_2O results in the operation of the body's osmolality regulating mechanisms.

Osmoreceptors

Alterations of the plasma osmolality are detected by *osmoreceptors* in the vicinity of the supraoptic and paraventricular areas of the hypothalamus, which are supplied with blood by the internal carotid artery. These receptors regulate the release of the hormone ADH (antidiuretic hormone, vasopressin). These receptors, and others in the lateral preoptic area of the hypothalamus, also affect thirst.

The addition to the body fluid of excess water lowers the plasma osmotic pressure, i.e. the solutes are diluted. Water deficiency, in contrast, increases the plasma osmotic pressure. These changes lead to an appropriate change in ADH release (Figure 7.1).

The functional characteristics of the osmoreceptors can be seen in Figure 7.2; the relationship between the plasma osmolality and the plasma ADH concentration is such that at normal plasma osmolality (i.e. about 285 mosmoles/kg H_2O) there is ADH present in the plasma; lowering the plasma osmolality reduces the ADH concentration and raising the plasma osmolality increases the plasma ADH concentration. The effect of changing plasma ADH concentrations on the urinary osmolality is shown in Figure 7.3. This coupling of the ADH-sensitive concentrating mechanism to the precise control of ADH release by osmoreceptors provides a very good regulatory mechanism for plasma osmolality.

The Sensitivity of the Osmoreceptors to Osmotic Changes Caused by Different Solutes

Normally, sodium and its associated anions contribute over 95 per cent of the osmotically active constituents of the plasma, and where osmotic changes are brought about by loss or gain of water in the body, the Na^+ concentration will be altered. However, addition or loss of solutes unaccompanied by water also changes plasma osmolality

Figure 7.1: The regulation of osmolality by ADH.

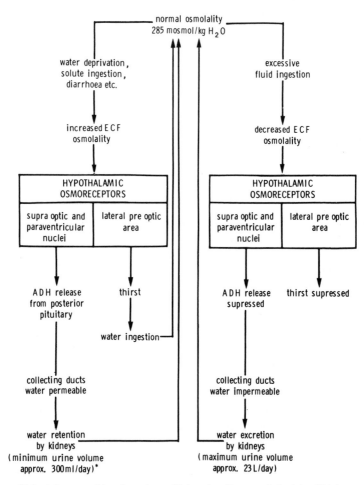

*the minimum possible urine volume will depend on the amount of solute which has to be excreted, since the maximum urine concentration is about 1400 mosmoles/Kg H_2O. See fig. 7.3.

(as will be discussed in more detail in the following chapter), and not all solutes are equally effective osmoreceptor stimulants. Their effectiveness depends on the degree to which they are unable to cross cell membranes (i.e. their ability to cause cellular dehydration).

Figure 7.2: ADH release from the posterior pituitary alters when plasma osmolality changes. If the plasma osmolality increases, ADH release increases to raise the plasma ADH level. Decreases of plasma osmolality reduce the plasma ADH level.

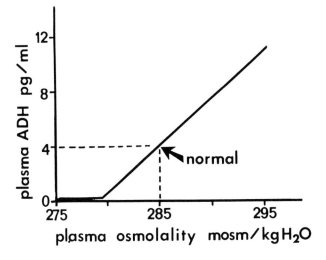

Synthesis and Storage of ADH

Antidiuretic hormone is synthesised primarily in the supraoptic nucleus of the hypothalamus. It is a nonapeptide if the sulphur-containing amino acids are regarded as two linked cysteine residues (or an octapeptide if they are regarded as a single cystine residue). The molecular weight is just over 1,000, and the structure of human ADH is

Cys-Tyr-Phe-Glutamide-Aspartamide-Cys-Pro-Arg-Gly(NH$_2$)

$$\underset{}{\Big\lfloor\!\!\rule{0pt}{0pt}\underline{\quad\quad S\quad\quad\quad\quad S\quad\quad\quad}\!\!\Big\rfloor}$$

This is generally termed 8-arginine-vasopressin, to distinguish it from the antidiuretic hormone found in pigs and some other species, where the arginine residue is replaced by lysine to form 8-lysine-vasopressin.

The hormone, after synthesis, is transported from the hypothalamus to the neurohypophysis (posterior pituitary) within nerve fibres which constitute the hypothalamo-hypophyseal nerve tract. For this transport process, ADH is associated with a larger protein molecule (neurophysin, M.Wt about 10,000) and the movement along the nerve axons occurs at a rate of 1-2 mm/day. The ADH-neurophysin granules are stored in

Figure 7.3: The relationship of plasma ADH concentration to urine osmolality. A tenfold change in plasma ADH concentration (from 0.5 to 5 pg/mℓ) is responsible for almost the full range of urine osmolalities.

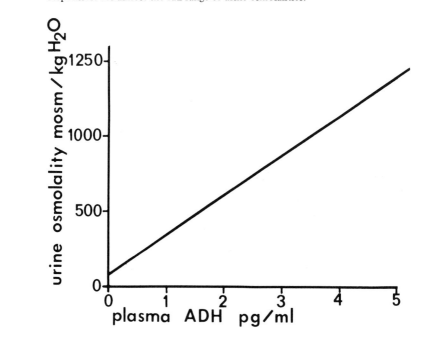

nerve terminals in the neurohypophysis.

Cellular Actions of ADH on Water Permeability

ADH only increases water permeability when it is present on the peritubular side of the collecting tubule cell, and is ineffective from the luminal side. This suggests that the ADH receptors are on the peritubular membrane of the tubule cells. The hormone-receptor complex then activates the enzyme adenyl cyclase, which catalyses the formation of cyclic 3'5'-AMP (adenosine monophosphate) from ATP. The cyclic AMP thus generated activates a further enzyme, protein kinase, which phosphorylates proteins in the luminal membrane of the tubule and so increases the water permeability.

Removal of ADH from the Blood

In order for ADH to regulate precisely the plasma osmolality, it is necessary not only that ADH should be rapidly released in response to dehydration and that the release is rapidly stopped when the dehydration is corrected, but also that ADH must be rapidly removed from the plasma. This removal occurs in the liver and in the kidney. Of the ADH removed from the plasma by the kidneys (about 50 per cent of the total), less than 10 per cent appears in the urine, the remainder being metabolised.

The plasma half-life of ADH (i.e. the time taken for the plasma ADH concentration to fall by 50 per cent) is 10-15 mins.

Drugs Affecting ADH Release

A number of pharmacological agents may alter ADH release and thereby disturb osmoregulation. Probably the most widely used drug which increases ADH release is nicotine. Other drugs with a similar effect include ether, morphine and barbiturates. Conversely, some drugs – notably alcohol – inhibit ADH release.

The Regulation of Water Excretion and Water Reabsorption

When the body fluids have become hypertonic (e.g. because of dehydration), the function of the kidneys is to reabsorb 'pure' (i.e. osmotically 'free') water from the tubular fluid, to dilute the plasma. In the process, the urine becomes concentrated. Conversely, if excess water has been ingested, the function of the kidney is to excrete this excess 'pure' (osmotically 'free') water, so that dilute urine is produced. Thus, in the production of concentrated urine, osmotically-free water is reabsorbed, whereas in the production of dilute urine, osmotically-free water is excreted. (Note that 'dilute' urine has a lower osmolality than plasma and 'concentrated' urine has a higher osmolality than plasma.)

Whether the kidneys produce dilute or concentrated urine depends primarily on the level of circulating ADH, since changes in ADH levels affect not only the volume of urine excreted, but also the urinary concentration. This is because, although ADH has little effect on the quantity of solute excretion, the volume of water in which the solutes are excreted is altered by ADH.

If the kidney is producing urine which is isotonic to the plasma, then the osmotically-active constituents of the urine are being excreted in a volume of water sufficient to keep the solutes at the same osmotic pressure as the plasma. This volume of water, in mℓ/min, is the rate at which osmotically-active substances are cleared from the plasma, i.e. is the osmolar clearance. We can define osmolar clearance using the clearance formula (p. 79) as

osmolar clearance, $C_{osm} = \dfrac{U_{osm}\ V}{P_{osm}}$

where U_{osm} and P_{osm} are, respectively, the urine and plasma osmolalities, and V is the urine flow (ml/min). In the case cited above, of the urine being isotonic to the plasma, then

$$\frac{U_{osm}}{P_{osm}} = 1$$

so $C_{osm} = V$

If the urine osmolality is lower than the plasma osmolality, i.e. if dilute urine is being produced, then, since U_{osm}/P_{osm} is less than 1, C_{osm} must be less than V. Another way of saying this is that the urine volume per minute, V, is made up of an additional volume of 'free' water (C_{H_2O}) as well as isotonic fluid (C_{osm}). So:

$$V = C_{osm} + C_{H_2O}$$

where C_{H_2O} is the free-water clearance. Free water is excreted when ADH levels are low (so that the urine is dilute); the excretion of free water raises the plasma osmolality, P_{osm}. The excretion of free water depends on (a) the generation of osmotically-free water in the ascending limb of the loop of Henle by NaCl absorption unaccompanied by water, and (b) the excretion of this osmotically-free water because of the impermeability of the collecting ducts, preventing its reabsorption. The maximum C_{H_2O} in man is 12-15 ml/min (15-22 l/day).

If the urine osmolality is greater than the plasma osmolality (i.e. if concentrated urine is being produced) then U_{osm}/P_{osm} is greater than 1, and V must be less than C_{osm}. So in the equation

$$V = C_{osm} + C_{H_2O}$$

C_{H_2O} must be negative. However, it is rather confusing to speak of negative free-water clearance — what this really means is that free water is being absorbed, not excreted. So we can introduce the term 'free water reabsorption', $T^c_{H_2O} = -C_{H_2O}$

and $V = C_{osm} - T^c_{H_2O}$

so $T^c_{H_2O} = C_{osm} - V$

For example, suppose that $V = 1$ mℓ/min, $P_{osm} = 290$ mosmoles/kg and $U_{osm} = 1,000$ mosmoles/kg. Then

$$C_{osm} = \frac{U_{osm}.\ V}{P_{osm}} = \frac{1000}{290} \times 1 = 3.45 \text{ m}\ell/\text{min}$$

$$\begin{aligned} \text{and } T^c_{H_2O} &= C_{osm} - V \\ &= 3.45 - 1 \\ &= 2.45 \text{ m}\ell/\text{min} \end{aligned}$$

This 2.45 mℓ/min is the volume of solute-free water being returned to the plasma by renal absorption.

In circumstances in which there is solute-free water reabsorption, free water is still generated in the ascending limb of the loop of Henle, but this (and more) is reabsorbed during the passage of the tubular fluid along the collecting tubules, so that the final urine is more concentrated than the plasma.

Measurements of C_{H_2O} and $T^c_{H_2O}$ are quantitative ways of determining the ability of the kidney to excrete or conserve water. They are also useful measurements to indicate the physiological sites of action of diuretics (see Chapter 14).

The Effect of Solute Output on Urine Volume

Because the concentrating ability of the kidneys is limited (maximum urinary osmolality is about 1,400 mosmoles/kg), it follows that the amount of urine excreted per day can depend not only on the level of circulating ADH, but also on the amount of solute to be excreted (Figure 7.4).

For example, suppose we have 800 mosmoles of solute to excrete per day. Since the maximum urinary osmolality is 1,400 mosmoles/kg H$_2$O, the *minimum* volume of urine which can be excreted is

$$\frac{800}{1,400} \text{ kg H}_2\text{O}/24 \text{ hrs} = 592 \text{ m}\ell/24 \text{ hrs (point a, Figure 7.4)}$$

If the amount of solute to be excreted per day were 2,000 mosmoles, then the *minimum* volume of urine which can be excreted is

$$\frac{2,000}{1,400} \text{ kg H}_2\text{O}/24 \text{ hrs} = 1,430 \text{ m}\ell/24 \text{ hrs (point b, Figure 7.4)}$$

Thus the excretion of large amounts of solute causes a diuresis, even in the presence of high levels of ADH.

From the foregoing, it should be apparent why it is not possible

Figure 7.4: The effect of ADH on urine output. Since ADH enables urine to be concentrated by water abstraction from the collecting ducts, the urine in the presence of maximal ADH has an osmolality of about 1,400 mosmoles/kg H_2O. However, the amount of urine produced per day, of this osmolality, will depend on the amount of solute to be excreted. Point a shows the minimum possible urine output with a solute excretion of 800 mosmoles/24 hrs, whereas point b shows the minimum urine output if 2,000 mosmoles/24 hrs have to be excreted.

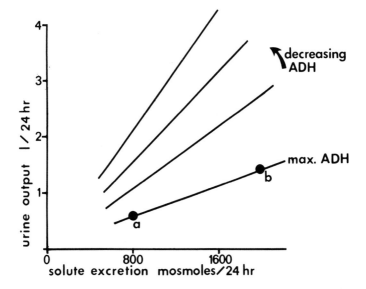

for man to survive by ingesting very hypertonic solutions. Suppose that a subject ingests 1 litre of a 2,000 mosmoles/kg H_2O solution. Since the maximum urine osmolality is 1,400 mosmoles/kg H_2O, the excretion of this solute cannot occur in less than

$$\frac{2,000}{1,400} \text{ kg } H_2O = 1,430 \text{ m}\ell$$

Thus more water is required to excrete the solute than was ingested with it, and the subject becomes dehydrated.

Some non-reabsorbable solutes, such as mannitol, impair the renal concentrating ability and lead to the production of an almost isotonic urine. Such solutes are termed 'osmotic diuretics' and are fully discussed in Chapter 14.

Adrenal Steroids and the Renal Response to ADH

Adrenal insufficiency impairs the renal response to water loading, i.e. very dilute urine cannot be produced. In the absence of adrenal steroids (glucocorticoids), the collecting duct water permeability is above the basal level, even in the absence of ADH, and the effect of ADH on permeability appears to be reduced.

Suggestions for Further Reading

Dousa, T.P. and H. Valtin. 'Cellular actions of vasopressin in the mammalian kidney', *Kidney Int., 10* (1976), pp. 46-63

Dunn, F.L., T.J. Brennan, A.E. Nelson and G.L. Robertson. 'The role of blood osmolality and volume in regulating vasopressin secretion in the rat', *J. Clin. Invest., 52* (1973), pp. 3212-19

Hammer, M., J. Ladefoged and K. Ølgaard. 'Relationship between plasma osmolality and plasma vasopressin in human subjects', *Am. J. Physiol., 238* (1980), pp. E313-17

Pollock, A.S. and A.I. Arieff. 'Abnormalities of cell volume regulation and their functional consequences', *Am. J. Physiol., 239* (1980), pp. F195-205

Robertson, G.L., R.L. Shelton and S. Athar. 'The osmoregulation of vasopressin', *Kidney Int., 10* (1976), pp. 25-37

Zimmerman, E.A. and A.G. Robinson. 'Hypothalamic neurones secreting vasopressin and neurophysin', *Kidney Int., 10* (1976), pp. 12-24

8 THE REGULATION OF BODY FLUID VOLUME

Introduction

Sodium salts are the main osmotically active solutes of the extra-cellular fluid (ECF). Thus, since body fluid osmolality is regulated by osmoreceptors and ADH release, if the extracellular fluid sodium content changes, then ECF volume will also change (Figure 8.1).

It follows that the regulation of ECF volume (and indirectly, of total body fluid) is brought about by the regulation of the body sodium content. This control of body sodium content is a vital function of the kidneys. In order to understand how this control is effected, we must introduce the concept of 'effective circulating volume'.

'Effective Circulating Volume'

Changes in the extracellular fluid Na^+ content, because they change the ECF volume, will affect the volume of blood perfusing the tissues. The 'effective circulating volume' is the component of the ECF which is perfusing the tissues. It should be noted that the effective circulating volume is not necessarily identical to the intravascular (blood) volume, since there may be circumstances in which not all of the blood is effect-ively perfusing the tissues (see Chapter 13).

When osmotic changes occur in the body, the response (increased or decreased ADH release) takes place within minutes, and the disturbance is rapidly corrected. In contrast, disturbances in body sodium content (and, consequently, in body fluid volume) may take many hours, or even days, to correct.

The maintenance of the body fluid volume depends on an adequate sodium intake. In the dog, if sodium is completely excluded from the diet, losses from the body (via the skin and kidneys) occur at the rate of about 25 mmoles of Na^+ per day. And, because osmoregulation occurs, there is a gradual reduction in the body fluid volume (this reduction is primarily of ECF volume). Man is able to conserve sodium more effectively than the dog, and the urine can be almost free of sodium (urinary Na^+ can be less than 1 mM). However, this maximal sodium reabsorption can affect the excretion of K^+ and H^+, and so may disturb acid-base balance — see Chapter 9.

Theoretically, it would be possible for sodium excretion to be

Figure 8.1: The presence of an osmoregulatory mechanism means that changes in ECF sodium *content* will change the ECF volume (so that ECF sodium *concentration* stays constant).

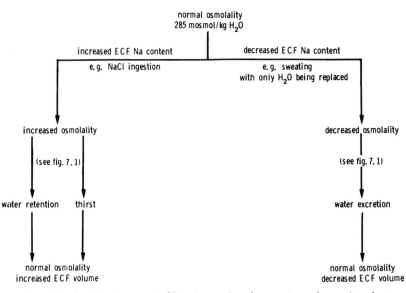

altered either by changes in filtration or by changes in reabsorption, but the amount filtered probably does not change significantly (except transiently) in man under physiological conditions, and changes in Na^+ excretion are normally brought about by changes in tubular reabsorption. (However, although the amount filtered stays relatively constant, the distribution of filtration between different nephrons may change.)

Exactly how Na^+ reabsorption is modified by changes in ECF volume (and effective circulating volume) is still a matter of some debate. In fact it probably constitutes the major unsolved problem in renal physiology at the present time. Nevertheless, many facts are clear and we can therefore attempt to integrate these facts in a coherent story of how Na^+ reabsorption is regulated.

Aldosterone

If the adrenal glands are removed, a number of metabolic defects appear and, in most species, death occurs within about two weeks. The cause of death is generally the loss of NaCl from the body leading to circulatory collapse. There is excessive NaCl (and very little K^+) in the urine and the plasma sodium concentration falls (whereas the plasma potassium concentration increases). These changes lead to the movement of K^+ (and water) into the cells so that the intracellular fluid volume increases. The ECF volume is therefore markedly decreased because of NaCl and water loss in the urine and the movement of water into the cells.

The above changes are due to the absence of the adrenal cortical hormone, *aldosterone*. Death can usually be postponed, after removal of the adrenal glands, either by a high sodium diet (to maintain ECF volume in spite of the urinary loss of NaCl and water), or by the administration of aldosterone.

It is thus apparent that *aldosterone is necessary for normal sodium reabsorption to occur*. However, this does not necessarily mean that aldosterone regulates Na^+ excretion; only that aldosterone is necessary for such regulation to occur, i.e. aldosterone has a *permissive action*, permitting Na^+ regulation. This caution in interpreting the role of aldosterone in Na^+ regulation is necessary because, when there are abnormalities in the secretion of aldosterone, Na^+ reabsorption and excretion, and thus regulation of ECF volume, are often unimpaired.

Aldosterone stimulates Na^+ reabsorption from the distal convoluted tubule. The mechanism for sodium reabsorption at this site is loosely coupled (see p. 116) to H^+ and/or K^+ secretion. So, in promoting Na^+ reabsorption, aldosterone also promotes H^+/K^+ secretion. (Aldosterone also promotes Na^+ reabsorption from the colon and gastric glands, and from the ducts of sweat glands and salivary glands.)

Changes in plasma aldosterone levels usually lead to parallel changes in ADH levels, because increased sodium reabsorption leads to increased plasma osmolality, which (via the hypothalamic osmoreceptors) increases ADH secretion from the posterior pituitary, to promote water reabsorption from the collecting ducts. Together, the two hormones (aldosterone and ADH) can be considered as leading to the reabsorption of an isotonic absorbate which maintains the ECF volume.

However, when excess aldosterone is produced, or if aldosterone is administered in excess, sodium retention (and oedema) rarely occurs — i.e. there is an 'escape' mechanism, whereby sodium excretion returns to normal in spite of the abnormal aldosterone level. This phenomenon emphasises the complicated nature of body fluid volume regulation, and the fact that aldosterone cannot be said to be *the* regulator of sodium excretion.

Control of Aldosterone Release

Plasma K⁺ Concentration. Increases in plasma potassium concentration have a direct action on the adrenal cortex, stimulating aldosterone secretion. Very small changes in the plasma K^+ concentration (e.g. of 0.1 mM) can significantly increase aldosterone release. The consequence of this is increased distal tubular K^+ secretion, returning the plasma K^+ concentration to normal, so that aldosterone release decreases.

Plasma Na⁺ Concentration. Decreases in plasma sodium concentration have a direct effect on the adrenal cortex, to stimulate aldosterone secretion. However, this is *not* an important way in which aldosterone release is altered, because osmoregulation normally keeps the plasma sodium concentration constant.

Changes in the Extracellular Fluid Volume. Because of the osmoregulatory mechanism, decreases in the body sodium *content* lead to decreases in the effective circulating volume. Changes in the effective circulating volume alter aldosterone release via the renin-angiotensin system.

Renin and Angiotensin, and their Relationship to Aldosterone

Renin, the enzyme synthesised and stored in the juxtaglomerular apparatus, is released into the plasma when the body sodium content decreases. It is unlikely that the body sodium content can directly provide the stimulus for renin release; rather the stimulus must be some change brought about by altered body sodium content. As noted earlier, body sodium content determines the effective circulating volume and it is this relationship which determines renin release. Decreased effective circulating volume decreases the renal afferent-arteriolar pulse pressure. This change in pressure in the afferent arteriole is detected by the cells of the juxtaglomerular apparatus in the wall of the afferent arteriole, and renin release is stimulated. It has also been suggested that changes in distal tubular sodium (content or concentration) may be detected by the macula densa, and that this may also regulate renin release. However, it is not entirely clear how distal tubular sodium changes as a result of alterations in renal perfusion. (It has been suggested that a fall in the rate of delivery of sodium to the macula densa increases renin release, although very recently chloride rather than sodium has been implicated as the stimulus acting on the macula densa.)

Figure 8.2: The regulation of angiotensin II formation by body sodium content.

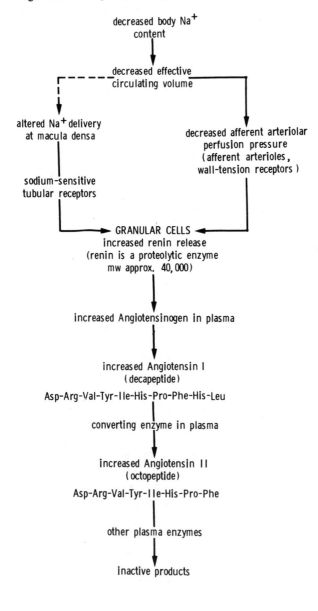

Following stimulation of the juxtaglomerular apparatus, renin is released into the blood, where it acts on a plasma protein (an $\alpha2$ globulin), angiotensinogen (also called 'renin substrate') and splits off a decapeptide, angiotensin I. An enzyme in the plasma, 'converting enzyme', rapidly removes a further two amino acids from angiotensin I, to form the octapeptide, angiotensin II (Figure 8.2). Angiotensin II is an extremely potent vasoconstrictor, and this action could be of great significance within the kidney (see below). However, angiotensin II also acts on the zona glomerulosa of the adrenal gland, to release aldosterone (Figure 8.3).

Aldosterone, in common with all adrenal cortical hormones, is synthesised from cholesterol, which may be synthesised within the gland or taken up from the circulation. (The structure of aldosterone is shown in Figure 14.2.) Very little aldosterone is stored. Stimuli to its release promote aldosterone biosynthesis.

In spite of the relationship between renin release and aldosterone, it is apparent from the 'escape' phenomenon that factors other than aldosterone can regulate sodium reabsorption. The vasoconstrictor properties of angiotensin II may be important in this respect, as will become clear from the following section.

The third action of angiotensin II (Figure 8.3) is the stimulation of thirst. This is a direct action of angiotensin II on the brain.

Figure 8.3: Actions of angiotensin II.

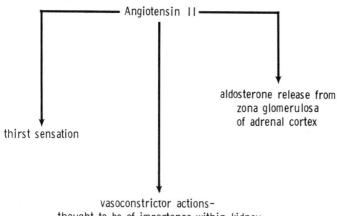

aldosterone release from
zona glomerulosa
of adrenal cortex

thirst sensation

vasoconstrictor actions–
thought to be of importance within kidney

Starling Forces and Proximal Tubular Sodium Reabsorption

When the body sodium content changes, the modifications of effective circulating volume which result, *automatically* adjust proximal tubular sodium reabsorption in the direction required to correct the disturbance. We saw in Chapter 4 that the uptake of sodium chloride from the lateral intercellular spaces of the proximal tubule into the capillaries depends on Starling forces. These forces therefore determine net sodium chloride reabsorption in the proximal tubule.

The rate of uptake of sodium chloride and water from the proximal tubule into the peritubular capillaries is determined by the rate of uptake from the lateral intercellular spaces into the capillaries; this rate of uptake is shown by the equation:

capillary uptake $\propto$ forces favouring uptake − forces opposing uptake

$$\propto (\Pi_{cap} + P_{LIS}) - (\Pi_{LIS} + P_{cap})$$

where Π is oncotic pressure, P is hydrotatic pressure, LIS is lateral intercellular space and cap is capillary.

Both the peritubular capillary hydrostatic pressure and the plasma protein osmotic pressure (oncotic pressure) are altered by changes in body fluid volume. Increases in volume (caused, for example, by increased NaCl and water content of the body), result in increased peritubular capillary hydrostatic pressure and, at the same time, dilute the plasma proteins and hence reduce the oncotic pressure. These changes decrease proximal tubular reabsorption of NaCl and water, and so increase the delivery of NaCl and water to more distal parts of the nephron.

The increased peritubular capillary hydrostatic pressure in such circumstances is due to an increased *venous pressure* (caused by increased circulating volume), rather than the transmission of an increased arterial pressure to the capillaries.

But although proximal tubular NaCl and water reabsorption are automatically adjusted to the requirements of the body for sodium excretion or sodium conservation, changes in proximal sodium reabsorption are not necessarily reflected in the final urine. This is because NaCl reabsorption in the ascending limbs of long loops of Henle is directly dependent on NaCl delivery. Reduced proximal NaCl reabsorption will increase the delivery of NaCl to the ascending limbs, where more NaCl will be extruded into the medullary interstitium. So it might appear that the loops of Henle are 'sabotaging' the efforts of the proximal tubules to correct volume disturbances. However, the nephrons with short loops of Henle may not transport a sufficient amount of NaCl out of the ascending limbs to reabsorb all of the excess if the delivery from the proximal tubule increases. We could thus term the short-looped nephrons 'sodium-losing nephrons', and the long-looped nephrons 'sodium-retaining nephrons'. The final urinary composition of the short-looped nephrons may depend on proximal reabsorption to a much greater extent than that of the long-looped nephrons. It should therefore be apparent that the effect of changes in proximal tubular NaCl and water reabsorption on the final urine could depend on the contribution to urine formation of the two types of nephrons.

Redistribution of Filtration amongst the Nephron Population

There is evidence (somewhat controversial) that in rats on a low sodium diet, filtration is lower in the cortical glomeruli than in juxtamedullary ones. In rats on a high sodium diet, the ratio is reversed, cortical glomeruli having the higher GFR. It is not only GFR but blood flow to the different types of nephron which is affected.

The high sodium diet presents the need to excrete sodium, and hence the distribution of filitration could be directed to the superficial (short loops of Henle) nephrons, and vice versa on the low sodium diet. It is possible that this distribution of blood flow to the two types of nephron according to the need for sodium excretion or sodium conservation, may be mediated by the intrarenal haemodynamic actions of angiotensin II, although this is a controversial topic at the time of writing.

Renal Nerves

The activity in the renal sympathetic nerves is regulated by arterial baroreceptors. Increased body fluid volume will tend to increase blood pressure (b.p.), causing a reflex response mediated by the baroreceptor mechanism:

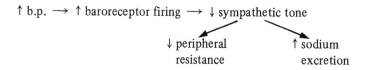

$\uparrow$ b.p. $\longrightarrow$ $\uparrow$ baroreceptor firing $\longrightarrow$ $\downarrow$ sympathetic tone

$\downarrow$ peripheral resistance $\uparrow$ sodium excretion

Conversely, decreases in body fluid volume, because they decrease the effective circulating volume, will tend to decrease blood pressure, which will reflexly (via the baroreceptors) increase sympathetic tone.

How do changes in the activity in the renal sympathetic nerves affect sodium excretion? The sympathetic nerves to the kidney go primarily to the afferent arterioles, and mild stimulation of the renal nerves reduces the blood flow to the superficial nephrons and increases blood flow to the juxtamedullary nephrons, which, as we saw in the previous section, could lead to sodium conservation. This effect of the renal nerves may be mediated by angiotensin II, because renal nerve stimulation is known to release renin. This will also cause sodium retention by leading to aldosterone release, but, in addition, there is some evidence that catecholamines released from the renal sympathetic nerve endings (and from the adrenal medulla) stimulate sodium reabsorption by the proximal tubule, though whether this is a direct action on sodium transport, or is due to altered peritubular forces, is a matter of conjecture at present. There is some evidence that the action is a direct one, since it has been demonstrated in isolated perfused renal tubules.

Prostaglandins

Prostaglandins are complex lipid molecules, which are synthesised in most cells of the body. In the kidney, there are at least three distinct sites of synthesis; these are (1) the cortex (including glomeruli), (2) medullary interstitial cells and (3) the collecting duct epithelial cells. The main prostaglandins synthesised by the kidney are PGE_2, PGI_2, $PGF_{2\alpha}$ and PGD_2.

Prostaglandins affect sodium and water excretion by the kidneys. Inhibition of renal prostaglandin biosynthesis (using a prostaglandin synthetase inhibitor such as aspirin or indomethacin) leads, in most experimental circumstances, to decreases in urine flow and sodium excretion, whereas renal arterial infusion of prostaglandins causes diuresis and natriuresis.

These actions of the renal prostaglandins are now quite well established, but their causes are still a matter of great controversy. Until recently it was thought that the urinary changes brought about by prostaglandins or prostaglandin synthetase inhibitors were due to changes in renal haemodynamics (prostaglandins of the E series are vasodilators), but many reports of the last year or two have indicated that prostaglandins are diuretic and natriuretic even when renal haemodynamics do not change, and this suggests that the renal prostaglandins have direct actions on renal tubular reabsorption. However, there is also evidence that the renal prostaglandins play a part in maintaining the renal blood flow in circumstances in which the renal blood supply is threatened (e.g. hypovolaemia).

Other Factors which may be Involved in Regulating Sodium Excretion

Kinins are vasodilator peptides produced from precursor proteins ('kininogens') by the enzyme kallikrein. Kinins are natriuretic, but their significance in the overall control of sodium excretion is not clear. The presence of both kallikrein and kinins can be demonstrated in the kidney. There is also a possibility that there is an as yet unidentified 'natriuretic hormone' released during volume expansion or in circumstances where the number of functioning nephrons is reduced, so that the remaining ones must increase the fraction of filtered sodium which they excrete.

ADH and the Relationship between Osmotic Regulation and Volume Regulation

In the previous chapter, it was seen that ADH release is controlled by osmoreceptors, and that changes in ADH release lead to changes in water reabsorption by the kidney, and thereby regulate body fluid osmolality. However, there are circumstances in which the maintenance of effective circulating volume is more important (to survival) than is the maintenance of body fluid osmolality. So when the effective circulating volume is threatened, volume regulation takes precedence over osmotic regulation. This is easily demonstrated: the diuresis brought about by water ingestion (i.e. decreased plasma osmolality) is greatly reduced by a small, non-hypotensive haemorrhage.

Changes in effective circulating volume are detected by stretch receptors in the right and left atria (afferent fibres are in the vagus nerve) and rapidly lead to appropriate alterations in urine flow (e.g. stretching the left atrial receptors produces a diuresis), probably mediated by changes in ADH release (although there are some suggestions that another, unknown, hormone may be involved). In addition to these receptors in the low-pressure parts of the circulation, receptors which can alter ADH release also exist in the arterial (high-pressure) part of the vascular system, and it is likely that these are activated by volume reductions which lead to blood pressure decreases.

How do body fluid osmolality and effective circulating volume

Figure 8.4: The effects of changes in body fluid volume on the regulation of body fluid osmolality by ADH. The black dots on each line show the normal plasma level of ADH for a particular body fluid volume. Thus, decreases in volume cause an adjustment, downwards, in the 'normal' osmolality – the body 'accepts' a lower osmolality (i.e. retains water) in order to minimise the decrease in volume.

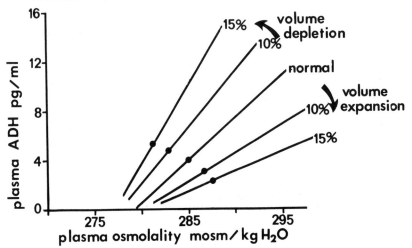

interact to regulate ADH release? Changes in volume alter the range of plasma osmolaities over which ADH is released, as shown in Figure 8.4. Put another way, decreases in effective circulating volume lead to increased ADH release to retain water, and this leads to a decreased plasma osmolality, so that the body accepts a reduced osmolality as the price for maintaining volume at a level higher than it otherwise would be.

It is important to realise that this control over ADH release by volume changes constitutes an 'emergency' mechanism, and that the main control over ADH is via osmoreceptors.

Overall Scheme of Body Fluid Volume Regulation

The obvious point which emerges from the foregoing discussion is that no *single* factor can be said to regulate sodium ion excretion. Instead many factors and mechanisms are involved, and this provides a 'fail-safe' system, whereby abnormalities or malfunctions affecting one factor are unlikely to disturb overall sodium balance.

For example, kidney transplantation is a widely performed operation,

Figure 8.5: The regulation of body fluid volume.

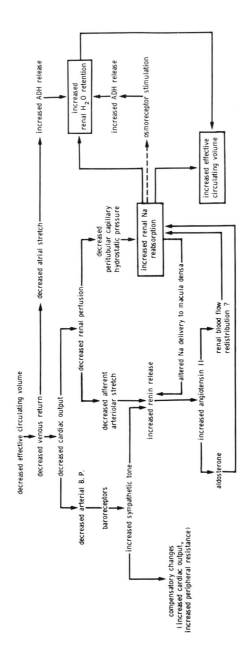

and transplanted kidneys are denervated. Nevertheless, they are able to maintain sodium balance and adjust sodium excretion according to the needs of the body. The fact that the renal nerves are not essential does not mean they have no function. If kidneys are denervated *in situ*, then a diuresis occurs (denervation diuresis) which usually lasts for some hours. This suggests that the nerves are normally playing a part in keeping urine flow (and sodium excretion) low, but that when the renal nerves are sectioned other control mechanisms can, after a time, compensate for the renal nerves.

Similar reasoning can be applied in the case of aldosterone. A certain minimum amount of aldosterone is necessary for life, but the absolute level is not critical for a steady state of sodium balance to be achieved.

In Figure 8.5 an attempt has been made to construct an integrated scheme of the main factors involved in the regulation of body fluid volume.

Suggestions for Further Reading

Claybaugh, J.R. and L. Share. 'Vasopressin, renin, and cardiovascular responses to continuous slow haemorrhage', *Am. J. Physiol.*, *224* (1973), pp. 519-23

Doyle, A.E., F.A.O. Mendelsohn and T.O. Morgan. *Pharmacological and Therapeutic Aspects of Hypertension*, vol. 1 (CRC Press, Boca Raton, Florida, 1980), pp. 1-13

Fitzsimons, J.T. *The Physiology of Thirst and Sodium Appetite* (Cambridge University Press, 1979)

Gauer, O.H., J.P. Henry and C. Behn, 'The regulation of extracellular fluid volume', *Annual Rev. Physiol.*, *32* (1970), pp. 547-95

Gill, J.R. 'Neural control of renal tubular sodium reabsorption', *Nephron, 23* (1979), pp. 116-18

Hermansson, K., M. Larson, Ö. Källskog and M. Wolgast. 'Influence of renal nerve activity on arteriolar resistance, ultrafiltration dynamics and fluid reabsorption', *Pflügers Archiv.*, *389* (1981), pp. 85-90

Knox, F.G., J.C. Burnett, D.E. Kohan, W.S. Spielman and J.C. Strand. 'Escape from the sodium retaining effects of mineralocorticoids', *Kidney Int.*, *17* (1980), pp. 263-76

Knox, F.G. and J.A. Diaz-Buxo. 'The hormonal control of sodium excretion' in S.M. McCann (ed.), *International Review of Physiology 16, Endocrine physiology II* (University Park Press, Baltimore, 1977), pp. 173-98

Robertson, G.L. and S. Athar. 'The interaction of blood osmolality and blood volume in regulating plasma vasopressin in man', *J. Clin. Endocrinol. Metab.*, *42* (1976), pp. 613-20

Stokes, J.B. and J.P. Kokko. 'Renal tubular sites of action of prostaglandins on salt transport' in A. Scriabine, A.M. Lefer and F.A. Kuehl (eds), *Prostaglandins in Cardiovascular and Renal Function* (MTP Press, Lancaster, 1980), pp. 425-38

9 THE RENAL REGULATION OF BODY FLUID pH

Introduction

In Chapter 1 it was pointed out that normal metabolism requires that the extra- and intracellular fluid compositions be kept relatively constant; this constancy includes pH. The pH must be maintained within fairly narrow limits — the normal blood pH is 7.40, and in health is kept within the range 7.35-7.45, although a range of 7.0-7.8 can be tolerated. But if the pH falls as low as 6.8, recovery is almost impossible.

It is not entirely clear why a pH of 7.4 is so important. Most of the enzyme reactions in the body have a pH optimum, but the pH-dependence of such reactions is much less sharply defined than the pH-dependence of the whole organism. However, by using the pH notation, we tend to obscure the range of variation of H^+ concentration which can be tolerated.* Thus the range of pH from 7.35 to 7.45 is an $[H^+]$ range of 45-35 nmol/litre, which is a change of over 20 per cent (it should be borne in mind that a 20 per cent change in, for example, body sodium concentration would have very serious consequences).

Physiological Buffers

A *buffer solution* is one which, when acid or base is added to it, minimises the change of pH. Buffer solutions consist of a weak acid and the conjugate base of that acid, i.e.

$$HA \; \rightleftharpoons \; H^+ \; + \; A^-$$
acid   proton   conjugate base

or, alternatively, the buffer solution may be a weak base and its conjugate acid:

$$B \; + \; H^+ \; \rightleftharpoons \; BH^+$$
base   proton   conjugate acid

---

* $pH = - \log [H^+]$, or, to put it another way, pH is the logarithm of the reciprocal of the H^+ concentration.

From the equations it is apparent that acids can donate protons, whereas bases can accept them. Several physiological buffers can be both acids and bases – they can accept or donate protons – and such substances are known as amphoteric. Amino acids and phosphate can behave in this way.

pK Values and Equilibrium Constants

The equilibrium for any reaction can be defined by an equilibrium constant, K. Thus for the reaction

$$HA \rightleftharpoons A^- + H^+$$

$$K = \frac{[H^+]\ [A^-]}{[HA]}$$

or in general terms $K = \dfrac{[H^+]\ [\text{base}]}{[\text{acid}]}$ (equation 1)

However, K is generally a very small figure, and it is therefore more convenient to use the term pK. This is analogous to pH, i.e. it is the log of $^1/K$.

$$\text{so} \quad pK = \frac{1}{\log K} = -\log K$$

$$\text{and} \quad pH = \frac{1}{\log [H^+]}$$

Then if we rearrange equation (1) above

$$H^+ = \frac{K.\ [\text{acid}]}{[\text{base}]}$$

we obtain what is known as the Henderson equation. Changing this into the pH and pK notation, we can derive

$$pH = pK + \log \frac{[\text{base}]}{[\text{acid}]}$$

which is known as the Henderson-Hasselbalch equation.

Table 9.1: The main physiological buffer systems.

Body Compartment	Buffer
blood	bicarbonate/CO_2
	haemoglobin (HHb/Hb^- and $HHbO_2/HbO_2^-$)
	plasma proteins ($H^+ \cdot Protein/Protein^-$)
	phosphate ($H_2PO_4^-/HPO_4^=$)
extracellular fluid	bicarbonate/CO_2
and CSF	proteins ($H^+ \cdot Protein/Protein^-$)
	phosphate ($H_2PO_4^-/HPO_4^=$)
intracellular fluid	proteins ($H^+ \cdot Protein/Protein^-$)
	phosphate ($H_2PO_4^-/HPO_4^=$)
	organic phosphates
	bicarbonate/CO_2

Source: Modified, with permission, from Gardner, M.L.G., *Medical Acid-base Balance: The Basic Principles* (Baillière Tindall, London, 1978).

Physiological Buffering

In the body fluids, there are several buffer systems (Table 9.1). In blood the main ones are the bicarbonate system, haemoglobin and the plasma proteins. Within the cells, the buffers include bicarbonate, phosphate and proteins. Throughout the body fluids, the bicarbonate buffer system is of primary importance. The reaction sequence for this system is:

$$CO_2 + H_2O \rightleftharpoons H_2CO_3 \rightleftharpoons H^+ + HCO_3^-$$

The great importance of this system stems from the precise regulation of the CO_2 concentration by the lungs, and the bicarbonate concentration by the kidneys. In fact, for the bicarbonate buffer system, we could simplify the Henderon-Hasselbach equation to:

$$pH \propto \frac{[HCO_3^-]}{pCO_2}$$

(where pCO_2 = partial pressure of CO_2, in mm Hg), and since bicarbonate is regulated by the kidneys and pCO_2 by the lungs, it is apparent that pH depends on the activity of both organs.

One further important point needs to be made before we consider how the renal regulation occurs. This point is that, by precisely fixing the [base]/[acid] ratio for one buffer system (the bicarbonate system), the pH of the body fluids is determined. This pH will then determine the [base]/[acid] ratio for all the other buffer systems in the body. The bicarbonate system, chemically, is a poor buffer, but physiologically it is extremely effective because of the control over $[HCO_3^-]$ and pCO_2.

The Renal Regulation of Plasma Bicarbonate Concentration

Table 9.2 shows the normal pCO_2, pH, $[H^+]$ and $[HCO_3^-]$ in the blood. It can be seen that bicarbonate is normally present in the plasma at a concentration of approximately 25 mM. Bicarbonate ion, HCO_3^-, is freely filtered at the glomeruli, hence the concentration of bicarbonate entering the nephron is also 25 mM. The kidney behaves *as if* there is a T_m for bicarbonate reabsorption (as shown in Figure 9.1) with the T_m * set very close to the amount which is filtered at the normal plasma concentration. This provides a means of dealing with increases in plasma $[HCO_3^-]$, since an increase will lead to the T_m being exceeded, and HCO_3^- being excreted until the plasma level is again too low to exceed the T_m.

Proximal Tubule

In the proximal tubule, most (90 per cent) of the filtered bicarbonate is absorbed from the tubular fluid. This bicarbonate reabsorption is in fact brought about not by the transport of HCO_3^- ions, but by the luminal conversion of HCO_3^- to CO_2 (Figure 9.2) Hydrogen (H^+) is actively secreted from the proximal tubule cell into the lumen, where it associates with HCO_3^- to form H_2CO_3. This carbonic acid dissociates into CO_2 and H_2O. The reaction is catalysed by an enzyme, *carbonic anhydrase*, which is present in the brush borders of the cells, and so catalyses the luminal reaction without being lost in the urine.

Table 9.2: Normal values for the bicarbonate buffer system in blood.

	$[H^+]$ (nmoles/ℓ)	pH	pCO_2 (mm Hg)	$[HCO_3^-]$ (mmoles/ℓ)
arterial	40	7.4	40	24
venous	46	7.35	46	25

* In fact the T_m for HCO_3^- is variable. It can be adjusted by the rate of H^+ secretion (see Chapter 4), but it also varies directly with the fractional sodium reabsorption.

Figure 9.1: The renal handling of HCO_3^-. There is an apparent T_m for HCO_3^- reabsorption, but this T_m is variable, as it depends primarily on the rate of tubular H^+ secretion. The limits of the variability are shown by the dashed lines. There is a similar degree of variability in the amount of HCO_3^- excreted at any particular filtered load, but for clarity this is not shown in the diagram.

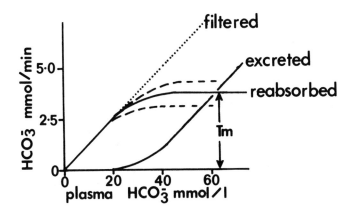

The CO_2 so formed can readily diffuse into the tubule cells, where intracellular carbonic anhydrase catalyses the rehydration of CO_2 to H_2CO_3, which dissociates to H^+ (available for secretion) and HCO_3^- which re-enters the plasma via the peritubular fluid. We might, therefore, claim that *the purpose of H^+ secretion is to permit HCO_3^- reabsorption.*

Although the entry of Na^+ into proximal tubular cells is passive (down the electrochemical gradient), the H^+ secretion process is active. However, Na^+ reabsorption and H^+ secretion are coupled, in the sense that they occur together to maintain electrical neutrality. (About 20 per cent of proximal sodium reabsorption is associated with H^+ secretion. The remainder occurs together with Cl^- absorption. For Na^+ associated with Cl^-, electrical neutrality is achieved by simultaneous, albeit passive, absorption of Cl^-.)

'Distal Tubule' and Collecting Duct

The fundamental acid-base regulating process that occurs in the 'distal tubule' and collecting duct is the same as that in the proximal tubule, viz. it is H^+ secretion. However, the process differs in a number of respects from that in the proximal tubule. The distal nephron processes are quantitatively much less important than those in the proximal tubule, since they account for only 10 per cent of the total bicarbonate

Figure 9.2: Proximal tubule HCO_3^- reabsorption. H^+, secreted into the lumen of the proximal tubule (left side of diagram), combines with filtered HCO_3^- to form carbonic acid (H_2CO_3), which is in turn rapidly converted to CO_2 and H_2O, catalysed by carbonic anhydrase. CO_2 which enters the cells can be rehydrated to carbonic acid, and hence can form HCO_3^- which enters the blood (right side of diagram). Thus CO_2 entry into the cells in this way is, in effect, HCO_3^- reabsorption. In the distal tubule, secreted H^+ can combine with luminal HCO_3^-, but there is no luminal carbonic anhydrase, hence there is little conversion of H_2CO_3 to CO_2 and H_2O, and so little bicarbonate reabsorption. In the distal tubule, secreted H^+ also combines with anions other than HCO_3^- (see Figures 9.3 and 9.4).

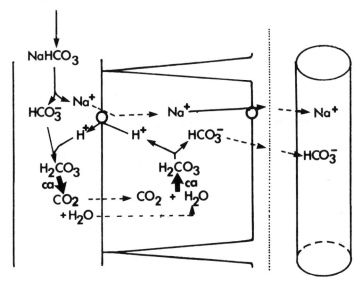

reabsorption. However, in order to achieve this, the distal tubule and collecting duct have to secrete H^+ against a much bigger gradient than that in the proximal tubule.

The 'distal tubule' secretes H^+ actively, in a loose exchange for reabsorbed Na^+, but the H^+ secretion appears to be to some extent competitive with the secretion of other cations, notably K^+. In the collecting duct, however, the secretion of H^+ occurs against such a steep concentration gradient that it seems likely there is an active H^+ secretion, tightly coupled to sodium reabsorption (i.e. a hydrogen-sodium exchange pump).

Although H^+ secretion distal to the loop of Henle reabsorbs the 10 per cent of filtered HCO_3^- which escaped reabsorption in the proximal tubules, it also has another function – the generation of further HCO_3^-

for the plasma. In order for H^+ secretion to occur, there must be some way in which the secreted H^+ can be 'mopped up' (i.e. buffered) in the tubular lumen, in order to provide a continuing gradient for secretion, or at least to prevent the gradient against which secretion is occurring from being too large. In the proximal tubule, it is mainly filtered HCO_3^- which does this H^+ buffering. In the distal nephron, there are other forms of combination for the secreted H^+.

Conversion of Alkaline Phosphate to Acid Phosphate

In the plasma there are two phosphate salts, disodium hydrogen phosphate (alkaline phosphate, Na_2HPO_4) and sodium dihydrogen phosphate (acid phosphate, NaH_2PO_4). The ratio alkaline phosphate:acid phosphate in plasma is approximately 4:1. This ratio is determined by the plasma pH according to the Henderson-Hasselbalch equation.

$$H^+ + HPO_4^= \rightleftharpoons H_2PO_4^-$$
proton base   acid

The pK for this reaction is 6.8, so

$$pH = 6.8 + \log \frac{[HPO_4^=]}{[H_2PO_4^-]}$$

and where pH = 7.4, the ratio $[HPO_4^=]/[H_2PO_4^-]$ is 4:1.

Both the acidic and basic forms of phosphate are filtered at the glomerulus and, because of H^+ secretion into the nephron, the ratio $[HPO_4^=]/[H_2PO_4^-]$ is reduced, i.e. alkaline phosphate is converted to acid phosphate. This will occur to some extent in the proximal tubule (since there is a small fall in pH of the tubular fluid proximally), but the main conversion will occur in the distal tubule. The process is shown diagrammatically in Figure 9.3. The $H_2PO_4^-$ constitutes the *titratable acidity* of the urine.

The important point about this is that the *secretion of H^+ generates HCO_3^- for the plasma.*

Ammonia Secretion

In the distal tubule cells, ammonia is produced as a result of the conversion of glutamine to glutamic acid and α-ketoglutarate. The generation of NH_3 within the cells provides a gradient for the passive diffusion of NH_3 into the tubule (and into the peritubular environment). In the tubular lumen, secreted NH_3 combines with secreted H^+, to form

Figure 9.3: Conversion of alkaline phosphate to acid phosphate in the tubular lumen. Secreted H⁺ in both the proximal and distal tubules combines with filtered alkaline phosphate (Na_2HPO_4), to convert it to acid phosphate (NaH_2PO_4). The intracellular production of H⁺ for secretion generates an HCO_3^- ion which enters the plasma.

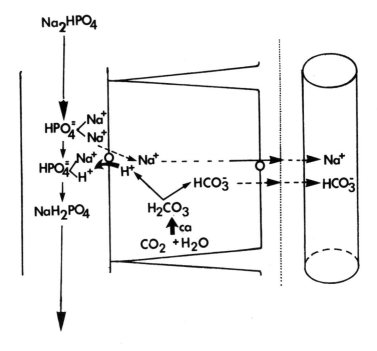

NH_4^+, which has a much lower permeance than NH_3, and is thus trapped in the tubular lumen and excreted (Figure 9.4).

The kidney is able greatly to increase NH_3 production, and hence NH_4^+ excretion; this in fact is one of the main ways in which the kidney responds to an acid load. And again, the *secretion of H⁺ generates HCO_3^- for the plasma.*

Summary

H⁺ secretion in the nephron leads to:

(1) bicarbonate reabsorption into the plasma;
(2) the generation of further bicarbonate to enter the plasma.

Figure 9.4: Secretion of NH_3 from distal tubular cells. NH_3 is manufactured within the cells by the deamination of glutamine to glutamic acid. NH_3 diffuses out of the cells in both directions (i.e. into the lumen and into the capillaries). H^+ secreted into the lumen combines with the secreted NH_3, converting it to NH_4^+, and ensuring that there is a concentration gradient for secretion of NH_3. Secretion of H^+ regenerates an HCO_3^- ion which enters the plasma.

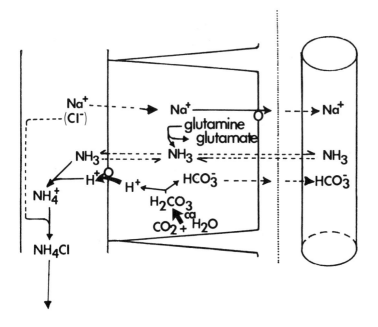

H^+ secretion demands that H^+ must be able to combine with anions in the tubule. For the process of bicarbonate reabsorption, the H^+ combines with bicarbonate itself. For the process of bicarbonate generation, the H^+ combines with $HPO_4^=$ or NH_3.

Because of H^+ secretion, the pH of the tubular fluid falls progressively along the nephron. This fall is small in the proximal tubule (from 7.40 down to about 6.90) but the pH may be as low as 4.5 in the collecting duct.

Although the urine is usually acidic and can be titrated to determine the 'titratable acidity', this only constitutes a fraction of the total H^+ secretion, because: total H^+ secretion $\equiv HCO_3^-$ reabsorption $+ H_2PO_4^=$ excretion $+ NH_4^+$ excretion; and only the $H_2PO_4^=$ excretion is 'titratable acidity'.

The Regulation of H⁺ Secretion According to Acid-base Balance Requirements

Acid-base disturbances can be divided into two categories, each with two sub-categories: (1) disturbances of respiratory origin: (i) respiratory acidosis and (ii) respiratory alkalosis; (2) disturbances of non-respiratory origin: (i) metabolic acidosis and (ii) metabolic alkalosis. (The term 'metabolic' refers to acid-base disturbances which affect the bicarbonate carbonic acid buffer system by a means other than an alteration of pCO_2. Such disturbances are frequently due to diet rather than metabolism *per se*.)

In each of the four disturbances, there is initially a change in body fluid pH (i.e. a change in H⁺ ion concentration). However, the buffer and compensatory systems are so effective that a change in pH may be barely measurable.

Changes in body fluid pH will include changes in arterial pH, and when changes in extracellular fluid pH occur, there are parallel (though not necessarily identical) changes in intracellular pH. Therefore a change in arterial pH is reflected in the pH of all the cells of the body, including the renal tubule cells. *The rate of H⁺ secretion from the tubule cells varies inversely with pH (i.e. varies directly with H⁺ concentration).* This is vital for the compensation for, and correction of, acid base disturbances.

Compensation vs Correction in Acid-base Disturbances

When an acid-base disturbance occurs, compensatory mechanisms immediately come into play to minimise and correct the pH change. However, these compensatory mechanisms do not restore acid-base balance to normal; they only restore pH to normal.

Normal acid-base status is not only a pH of 7.4, but is also a plasma [HCO₃⁻] of about 25 mM, and a plasma pCO_2 of about 40 mm Hg. An acid-base disturbance disturbs at least two of these three variables. *Compensation* is the restoration of pH *even though* [HCO₃⁻] and/or pCO_2 are still disturbed. *Correction* is the restoration of normal pH, [HCO₃⁻] and pCO_2. In fact, we might say that the purpose of the body's acid-balance regulating mechanisms is the maintenance of normal pH. The tools for this are pCO_2 and HCO₃⁻. The regulation of pCO_2 and [HCO₃⁻] *per se*, although of importance, is a subordinate function, which is sacrificed when necessary in the interests of pH regulation.

In the following pages, much use will be made of the graph of

Figure 9.5: Graph of plasma HCO_3^- concentration vs plasma pH for normal whole blood (i.e. plasma + red cells). pH, $[HCO_3^-]$ and pCO_2 are inter-related, and a knowledge of any two of the values enables us to determine the third. The point marked 'a' is the normal point – i.e. pH 7.4 (normal range 7.35–7.45), plasma $[HCO_3^-]$ 25 mM (normal range 24–27). pCO_2 40 mm Hg (normal range 35–48 mm Hg). In the following diagrams (Figure 9.6, 9.7, 9.8 and 9.9), point a is the normal point, point b is the uncompensated acid-base disturbance, and point c is an acid-base disturbance with compensation.

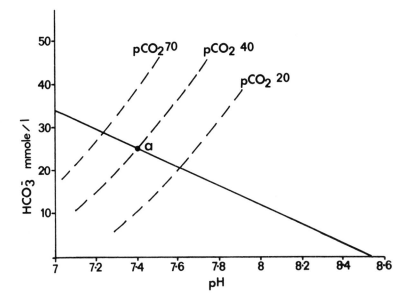

plasma HCO_3^- concentration vs plasma pH (Davenport, 1974). On this graph, pCO_2 isobars are shown (i.e. the partial pressure of CO_2, mm Hg), as in Figure 9.5. Because of the relationship between pH, HCO_3^- concentration and pCO_2 given by the equation

$$pH \propto \frac{[HCO_3^-]}{pCO_2}$$

if we know the value of any two of the variables, then there is only one possible value for the third variable, e.g. if we know pCO_2 and pH, there can be only one possible HCO_3^- concentration. The graph depicts this situation diagramatically.

Let us now examine the types of acid-base disturbance in detail. The distinction between 'compensation' and 'correction' should become clearer in the following sections.

In these sections, the simplified Henderson–Hasselbalch equation is used to show changes in pH, HCO_3^- and pCO_2, and three types of arrow are used to indicate changes:

$\blacktriangle$ or $\blacktriangledown$ is the initial acid-base defect
$\uparrow$ or $\downarrow$ is the consequence of the defect
$\overset{\shortmid}{\uparrow}$ or $\underset{\shortmid}{\downarrow}$ is compensation.

Respiratory Acidosis

This is a disturbance of acid-base balance which occurs when the respiratory system is unable to remove sufficient CO_2 from the body to maintain normal pCO_2. So the reaction is displaced to the right by the high pCO_2 (law of mass action):

$$CO_2 + H_2O \rightleftharpoons H_2CO_3 \rightleftharpoons H^+ + HCO_3^-$$

The *consequence* of this defect is an increased $[H^+]$ (i.e. reduced pH — acidosis), and an increased $[HCO_3^-]$. These changes are expressed graphically in Figure 9.6.

In the simplified form of the Henderson–Hasselbalch equation, we have:

$$\downarrow pH \propto \frac{[HCO_3^-] \uparrow}{pCO_2 \blacktriangle}$$

A change in $[H^+]$ in the body fluids changes the rate of H^+ secretion from renal tubular cells. In respiratory acidosis, $[H^+]$ is increased, therefore the rate of H^+ secretion also increases. This increased secretion is sufficient to reabsorb the filtered HCO_3^- (even though the plasma $[HCO_3^-]$ is raised by the defect, and therefore the amount of HCO_3^- filtered is increased) and to generate further HCO_3^- for the plasma. This increased renal H^+ secretion leading to increased plasma $[HCO_3^-]$ is the *compensation* for respiratory acidosis. It is shown graphically in Figure 9.6, and in the Henderson–Hasselbalch (simplified) equation below:

$$\overset{\shortmid}{\uparrow}\downarrow pH \propto \frac{[HCO_3^-] \uparrow \overset{\shortmid}{\uparrow}}{pCO_2 \blacktriangle}$$

Figure 9.6: Respiratory acidosis and its compensation. The defect in respiratory acidosis is an increase in the blood pCO_2, which increases the plasma $[HCO_3^-]$ and lowers the pH. These changes move the values of the three variables (pCO_2, pH, $[HCO_3^-]$) from the normal point a to point b.

Removal of the defect (i.e. a lowering of the pCO_2) would return $[HCO_3^-]$ and pH to normal. However, if the defect persists, then there is *compensation*, which serves to restore the pH towards normal. The compensation process is the renal retention of HCO_3^-, so that, on the graph, the values change from those of point b, to those of point c. Thus the defect (increased pCO_2) raises $[HCO_3^-]$, but compensation raises $[HCO_3^-]$ still further. This illustrates the important point that *it is pH which is regulated*. $[HCO_3^-]$ and pCO_2 are the 'tools' for the regulation of pH. (Generally, compensation occurs as the defect develops, so that the true change in the variables may occur along the line shown by the open arrow.)

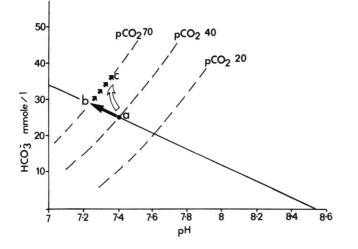

It should be noted that compensation restores the pH towards normal, but plasma $[HCO_3^-]$ is raised (both as a consequence of the defect, and by compensation), and pCO_2 is raised (the initial defect). To restore normal $[HCO_3^-]$ and pCO_2 would require a respiratory alteration, to lower pCO_2 (i.e. correction of the defect).

Respiratory acidosis (hypercapnia) is a pCO_2 of greater than about 45 mm Hg in arterial blood.

Causes of Respiratory Acidosis. The commonest causes of respiratory acidosis are chronic bronchitis and emphysema. Obstructions of the airway, for example by a foreign body, tumour or a constriction (in bronchial asthma), will also impair lung gas exchange and so raise arterial pCO_2, and mechanical injuries of the chest may impair respiration. Respiratory acidosis may also occur as a result of injuries and infections directly affecting the respiratory centre in the brain stem. General anaesthetics, morphine and barbiturates are respiratory centre depressants.

Other possible causes of respiratory acidosis include defective pulmonary diffusion (but this has a more marked effect on pO_2 than on pCO_2), and inadequate or non-uniform lung perfusion (although this too usually affects primarily the pO_2, and so may cause respiratory alkalosis — see below).

Respiratory Alkalosis

This is caused by the excessive removal of CO_2 from the body by the respiratory system, so that arterial pCO_2 falls below about 35 mm Hg. The reaction:

$$CO_2 + H_2O \rightleftharpoons H_2CO_3 \rightleftharpoons H^+ + HCO_3^-$$

is displaced to the left by the lowering of pCO_2, and this leads to a decrease in $[H^+]$ (i.e. a pH increase — alkalosis), and a decrease in $[HCO_3^-]$. The changes are shown graphically in Figure 9.7, and in the simplified Henderson-Hasselbalch equation we have

$$\uparrow pH \propto \frac{[HCO_3^-] \downarrow}{pCO_2 \quad \blacklozenge}$$

The decreased pCO_2 and consequent decreased $[H^+]$ in the renal tubule cells reduces the rate of H^+ secretion, so that, although the plasma $[HCO_3^-]$ is reduced, thereby reducing the amount of HCO_3^- filtered by the kidney, the rate of H^+ secretion is insufficient to reabsorb all the filtered bicarbonate, or to generate more bicarbonate. Thus HCO_3^- is excreted in the urine, and the plasma $[HCO_3^-]$ falls further.

The reduced H^+ secretion in the renal tubules, leading to HCO_3^- excretion, is renal *compensation* for respiratory alkalosis and is shown graphically in Figure 9.7. In the equation, we have:

$$\downarrow \uparrow pH \propto \frac{[HCO_3^-] \downarrow \downarrow}{pCO_2 \quad \blacklozenge}$$

The renal compensation restores pH to (or towards) normal, but it lowers the plasma $[HCO_3^-]$ (which was lowered anyway as a

Figure 9.7: Respiratory alkalosis and its compensation. The defect in respiratory alkalosis is decreased arterial pCO_2, which lowers the plasma $[HCO_3^-]$, and raises pH. Thus the values are shifted from point a to point b. The increased pH reduces the rate of renal H^+ secretion, so that less bicarbonate can be reabsorbed or regenerated by the kidney. This leads to compensation – i.e. the plasma $[HCO_3^-]$ falls, thereby lowering the pH towards normal (point c). If the defect develops slowly, the compensation will occur progressively as shown by the open arrow.

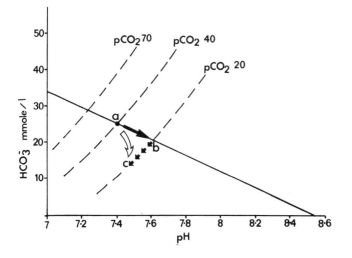

consequence of the defect) still further. pCO_2 is still reduced (the defect). The restoration of normal plasma $[HCO_3^-]$ and pCO_2 requires the removal of the respiratory defect – i.e. requires a reduction of ventilation.

Causes of Respiratory Alkalosis. Respiration serves to control the arterial pO_2 and pCO_2, and both oxygen and carbon dioxide partici- pate in the control of respiration. It is not appropriate in a renal physio- logy book to go into the control of respiration in detail; however, in order to understand the usual cause of respiratory alkalosis, some knowledge of respiratory control is essential.

Normally, the maintenance of an adequate pO_2 occurs automatically if respiration is adequate for the maintenance of normal pCO_2. In- creases in arterial pCO_2 increase H^+ concentration in most cells of the body, and this provides the stimulus (at brain-stem chemoreceptors) for an increased ventilation. Decreases in arterial pCO_2 decrease ventila- tion.

However, if the pO_2 in the inspired air is below normal, so that arterial pO_2 falls significantly, then oxygen lack, acting mainly via chemoreceptors in the carotid body, increases ventilation. When this occurs, the arterial pCO_2 falls. This is respiratory alkalosis.

So hypoxia, leading to increased respiration, can lead to hypocapnia and respiratory alkalosis. This occurs in normal people when they ascend to a high altitude (10,000 ft or more). Other causes of respiratory alkalosis include hyperventilation, which can be due to fever or brain-stem damage (affecting the pons), or to hysterical overbreathing.

Metabolic Acidosis

This is acidosis which is not caused by a change in the arterial pCO_2. So, in the reaction sequence

$$CO_2 + H_2O \rightleftharpoons H_2CO_3 \rightleftharpoons H^+ + HCO_3^-$$
$$\nwarrow_{H^+}$$

we can regard the metabolic acidosis as the addition of H^+ ions to the right of the reaction, so driving it to the left, and depleting the plasma HCO_3^- as it does so. (The direct loss of HCO_3^- will also cause metabolic acidosis — as will be clear from the Henderson-Hasselbalch equation below). Since respiration is unimpaired, we can consider that this sequence of events takes place initially at a constant (normal) pCO_2.

The acidosis is shown in Figure 9.8. In the equation, we have

$$\downarrow pH \propto \frac{[HCO_3^-] \quad \downarrow}{pCO_2}$$

The change in pH, acting on the central chemoreceptors, stimulates respiration, so that arterial pCO_2 falls. This is *respiratory compensation* for metabolic acidosis. However, the lowering of pCO_2 moves the reaction

$$CO_2 + H_2O \rightleftharpoons H_2CO_3 \rightleftharpoons H^+ + HCO_3^-$$

to the left thus lowering $[H^+]$ and so raising the pH towards normal, but also further lowering the plasma $[HCO_3^-]$ (Figure 9.8), i.e.

$$\uparrow \downarrow pH \propto \frac{[HCO_3^-] \quad \downarrow \downarrow}{pCO_2 \quad \downarrow \downarrow}$$

Figure 9.8: Metabolic acidosis and its compensation. Metabolic acidosis, the presence of excess H^+ in the body (from any source other than CO_2), can be regarded as occurring initially at a constant pCO_2. So in the development of metabolic acidosis, we move from point a to point b along the pCO_2 40 isobar. As explained in the text, plasma $[HCO_3^-]$ falls. The correction of the defect, to return from point b back to point a, occurs as a result of the renal excretion of the excess H^+. However, as it is obviously impossible for all of the excess H^+ to be excreted instantaneously, there is *respiratory compensation* for the metabolic acidosis. Acidosis stimulates the chemoreceptors in the medulla oblongata which control respiration, and brings about increased ventilation. This lowers the pCO_2, and also lowers plasma $[HCO_3^-]$, so we move from point b to a new point, c, by moving parallel to the normal HCO_3^-/pH line, in the direction of a lower pCO_2 isobar. Generally, the onset of a metabolic acidosis is immediately accompanied by respiratory compensation, so that the values of $[HCO_3^-]$, pH and pCO_2 change as shown by the open arrow.

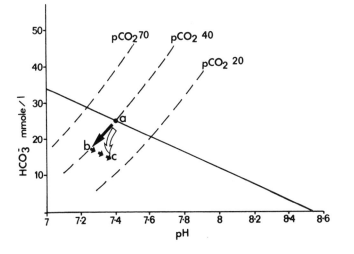

The removal of the defect is brought about because of the change in pH caused by the defect itself: the increased $[H^+]$ in the blood is reflected in an increased $[H^+]$ in the renal tubular cells, so that the rate of H^+ secretion is increased. This permits the reabsorption of all the filtered HCO_3^-, and the regeneration of more HCO_3^- so that the depleted plasma HCO_3^- is restored, thereby restoring the pH to normal, so that respiration can also be normalised.

Causes of Metabolic Acidosis. Metabolic acidosis can be caused by the ingestion of acids (H^+ ions), or the excessive metabolic production of

H^+, or the loss from the body of HCO_3^-.

It should be noted that, in metabolic acidosis, there is usually *nothing wrong* with the kidneys. They simply cannot excrete an H^+ load instantaneously. The respiratory compensation, by restoring pH towards normal, hampers the renal removal of the defect (i.e. the renal H^+ secretion and HCO_3^- reabsorption/regeneration). The exception to this is renal failure, where the kidneys' failure to excrete H^+ is the cause of metabolic acidosis (see Chapter 13).

Metabolic Alkalosis

This is alkalosis which is not caused by a change in the arterial pCO_2. In the reaction sequence

$$CO_2 + H_2O \rightleftharpoons H_2CO_3 \rightleftharpoons H^+ + HCO_3^-$$
$$\searrow\!\!\swarrow \qquad \diagdown OH^-$$
$$H_2O$$

we can regard metabolic alkalosis as the addition of base (OH^- in the equation, although it can be any H^+ acceptor) to the system, thereby removing H^+ from the right of the reaction and so causing the reaction to move to the right, increasing plasma $[HCO_3^-]$. We can regard this as occurring initially at a constant (normal) pCO_2 (Figure 9.9).

$$\uparrow \text{pH} \propto \frac{[HCO_3^-] \quad \uparrow}{pCO_2}$$

The decreased $[H^+]$, acting on central chemoreceptors, reduces ventilation and so increases the pCO_2. This is *respiratory compensation for metabolic alkalosis*.

$$\downarrow \uparrow \text{pH} \propto \frac{[HCO_3^-] \quad \uparrow \uparrow}{pCO_2 \quad \uparrow \uparrow}$$

The compensation brings down the pH, but further increases the plasma $[HCO_3^-]$.

The removal of the defect is brought about by the effect of the defect on renal H^+ secretion. The defect is decreased $[H^+]$ in the body, including the renal tubule cells, so the rate of H^+ secretion is reduced. This means that H^+ secretion is inadequate to reabsorb all the filtered HCO_3^- (or to generate more HCO_3^-), so the plasma $[HCO_3^-]$ falls, causing the reaction

Figure 9.9: Metabolic alkalosis and its compensation. Metabolic alkalosis, the loss of H^+ or addition of base to the body (for any reason other than a change in pCO_2), can be regarded as occurring initially at a constant pCO_2. So as metabolic alkalosis develops, we move from point a to point b along the pCO_2 40 isobar. Plasma $[HCO_3^-]$ increases (see text). The correction of the defect occurs as a result of a reduction in the rate of renal H^+ secretion. However, as this takes time to reduce the pH (and $[HCO_3^-]$), there is *respiratory compensation*. The increased pH, detected by the medulla oblongata chemoreceptors, reduces alveolar ventilation, and so increases the pCO_2 (and $[HCO_3^-]$). Thus we move from point b to point c, parallel to the normal pH/HCO_3^- line. As with metabolic acidosis, the onset of metabolic alkalosis brings the respiratory compensation into play immediately, so that the values of $[HCO_3^-]$, pH and pCO_2 change as shown by the open arrow.

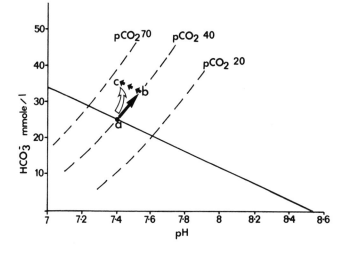

$$CO_2 + H_2O \rightleftharpoons H_2CO_3 \rightleftharpoons H^+ + HCO_3^-$$

to move to the right, restoring $[H^+]$ to normal.

As in the case of metabolic acidosis, the respiratory compensation hampers the renal removal of the defect. This fact again emphasises that it is the regulation of pH which is all important, rather than the regulation of $[HCO_3^-]$ or pCO_2 *per se*.

Causes of Metabolic Alkalosis. Metabolic alkalosis is most commonly caused by the loss of acid from the body by vomiting, thereby losing the hydrochloric acid from the stomach. Metabolic alkalosis is also caused by an increase of plasma bicarbonate. Changes in body fluid volume can alter plasma $[HCO_3^-]$, by altering the renal HCO_3^- threshold.

Suggestions for Further Reading

Davenport, H.W. *The ABC of Acid-base Chemistry*, 6th edn (University of
    Chicago Press, 1974)
Gardner, M.L.G. *Medical Acid-base Balance* (Baillière Tindall, London, 1978)
Kaehny, W.D. 'Pathogenesis and management of metabolic acidosis and alkalosis'
    in R.W. Schrier (ed.), *Renal and Electrolyte Disorders* (Little, Brown and Co.,
    Boston, 1976), pp. 79-120
—— 'Pathogenesis and management of respiratory and mixed acid-base
    disorders' in ibid., pp. 121-42
Pitts, R.F. 'The role of ammonia production and excretion in regulation of acid-
    base balance', *N. Engl. J. Med.*, *284* (1971), pp. 32-8
Rose, B.D. *Clinical Physiology of Acid-base and Electrolyte Disorders* (McGraw
    Hill, New York, 1977), pp. 165-210 and 295-376

10 RENAL CONTROL OF BODY FLUID POTASSIUM CONTENT

Introduction – the Importance of K^+ in the Body

In Chapter 7, the importance of Na^+ in the extracellular fluid was described and it was shown that the osmolality (of the extracellular fluid) depends on the body Na^+ content. Inside the cells, however, K^+ is the major cation, and the maintenance of K^+ balance is essential for life. The body contains 3-4 moles of K^+ (i.e. 120-160 g), but only about 2 per cent of this is extracellular. The normal cellular concentration of K^+ is 150-160 mmol/ℓ, whereas the normal plasma concentration is only 4-5 mmol/ℓ. The causes of this uneven distribution were discussed in Chapter 1.

The ratio intracellular $[K^+]$:extracellular $[K^+]$ affects the resting membrane potential of nerve and muscle cells, and hence affects their excitability. Hypokalaemia causes hyperpolarisation of the nerve and muscle cells (i.e. the resting potential becomes more negative), making the cells less sensitive to depolarising stimuli and therefore less excitable. Thus severe hypokalaemia can cause paralysis. Hyperkalaemia depolarises cells, making them more excitable, but in severe hyperkalaemia, the resting potential may be above (i.e. less negative than) the threshold potential, and this means that nerve cells are unable to repolarise after conducting an action potential, so that paralysis ensues.

Slow changes in the body K^+ content are much better tolerated than rapid changes. This is because, when the changes are slow, the equilibrium between intra- and extracellular potassium is maintained. Thus there may be hypokalaemia, but the ratio of $[K^+]$ intracellular: $[K^+]$ extracellular may be normal. In such circumstances, nerve and muscle cell excitability will also be normal.

The Regulation of Body K^+

A normal diet contains more than enough K^+ to satisfy the needs of the body, and hence the maintenance of K^+ balance is brought about by regulation of K^+ excretion. However, since the vast majority of K^+ ions in the body are intracellular, these intracellular 'stores' tend to buffer any changes in plasma $[K^+]$, i.e. a small decrease in plasma $[K^+]$ causes some movement of K^+ out of cells and hence the change in plasma $[K^+]$ is minimised. This implies that, for K^+ control to be effective, very small changes in plasma $[K^+]$ must be able to provide the stimulus for excretion to be adjusted.

Renal K ⁺ Handling

About 80 per cent of the filtered K^+ is reabsorbed proximally, and there is also some reabsorption in the loop of Henle. So much of the K^+ which is excreted appears in the tubular fluid by *secretion* from the distal tubule cells. The secretory process is thought to be passive, driven by the electrochemical gradient between the cells and the lumen. Na^+ absorption does to some extent determine the rate of K^+ secretion, but, in addition, any increase in the cellular $[K^+]$ will favour K^+ secretion, and any decrease in cellular $[K^+]$ will reduce K^+ secretion. This provides a means of automatically adjusting K^+ secretion to the body's requirements for K^+ balance.

Changes in distal tubular lumen $[K^+]$ influence the rate of K^+ secretion. Increases in the tubular $[K^+]$ decrease the rate of secretion, whereas decreases in the tubular $[K^+]$ increase the rate of K^+ secretion. The $[K^+]$ in the distal tubule, produced by a given rate of distal K^+ secretion, will be determined by the flow rate in the distal tubule. Thus diuretics (see Chapter 14) which increase distal tubular flow can increase the rate of K^+ secretion by lowering the tubular K^+ concentration (as well as by increasing Na^+ delivery to the distal tubule).

Aldosterone

Since the K^+-losing effects of aldosterone (see p. 100) do not exhibit the 'escape phenomenon' in the way that the Na^+-retaining effects do, there are good grounds for considering that, normally, aldosterone plays a more important role in determining K^+ balance than in regulating Na^+ excretion.

Until recently, it was thought that aldosterone regulated sodium-potassium exchange in the distal nephron in a stoichiometric manner. However, several studies have now shown that the aldosterone-sensitive transport mechanisms for sodium and potassium are independent of each other. The 'escape phenomenon' mentioned above is itself strong evidence for independent mechanisms for Na^+ and K^+, but in addition, the drug actinomycin D blocks the Na^+-retaining effects of aldosterone without inhibiting the K^+-losing effect, and, in adrenalectomised animals, very small amounts of aldosterone restore the plasma Na^+ concentration to normal, but do not significantly lower the elevated plasma K^+ concentration. This finding emphasises that, whereas for Na^+, aldosterone has a 'permissive action' (see Chapter 8), for K^+, aldosterone has a regulatory function.

Increases in plasma $[K^+]$ act directly on the adrenal cortex to increase aldosterone output, and decreases in plasma $[K^+]$ reduce aldosterone output. Aldosterone constitutes essentially the only hormonal control over K^+ output, whereas it is only one of many factors regulating Na^+ output.

Hypokalaemia

Since the diet almost invariably contains adequate K^+, hypokalaemia is generally due to losses of K^+ from the gastrointestinal tract, or by the kidneys. Persistent vomiting or diarrhoea, or the use of certain commonly prescribed diuretics (Chapter 14), are frequent causes of hypokalaemia.

The hypokalaemia in diarrhoea is due to the faecal loss of K^+ from the gastrointestinal secretions. Vomiting loses some K^+ directly in the vomitus, but the main effect of vomiting on K^+ balance is due to a change in urinary K^+ excretion. Vomiting causes metabolic alkalosis (due to the loss from the body of gastric HCl), and alkalosis reduces proximal tubular HCO_3^- absorption (Chapter 9), and also reduced proximal Na^+ absorption (since HCO_3^- stays in the tubule the associated cation – Na^+ – also stays in the tubule), and water absorption. The increased $NaHCO_3$ delivery to the distal tubule enhances Na^+ absorption at this site, and H^+ and K^+ are secreted in increased amounts. The increased tubular flow rate facilitates this. In addition, the loss of NaCl and volume depletion brought about by vomiting tends to increase aldosterone release from the adrenal cortex, which exacerbates the urinary K^+ loss.

Another relatively common cause of hypokalaemia is excess insulin (either exogenous insulin during diabetic treatment, or endogenous insulin). Insulin increases K^+ entry into cells (of skeletal muscle and liver), so that although the total amount of K^+ in the body is not altered directly, the extracellular $[K^+]$ decreases.

The physiological effects of a particular degree of hypokalaemia are widely different in different subjects. Most subjects remain symptom-free until plasma $[K^+]$ has fallen to approximately half its normal value (i.e. down to 2-2.5 mmol/ℓ). The initial symptom is muscle weakness, usually affecting the lower extremities, and gradually extending upwards, until death occurs when respiratory function becomes affected.

Potassium deficiency causes numerous other derangements of metabolism. The synthesis of liver and muscle glycogen requires potassium, so, since the conversion of glucose to glycogen is altered by hypokalaemia, the condition produces an abnormal glucose tolerance test. Hypokalaemia also affects vascular tone (causes vasoconstriction). Polyuria and thirst are present, because the renal response to ADH is impaired by hypokalaemia, so patients are unable to produce concentrated urine (see below). Metabolic alkalosis is frequently present in hypokalaemic patients, since the K^+ deficit tends to cause an increased intracellular $[H^+]$, which leads, in the distal tubule cells, to increased H^+ secretion. As the physiological effects of a particular degree of hypokalaemia are widely different in different subjects, it is best to assess the *functional* effects of hypokalaemia. This can be done by monitoring the ECG and muscle strength.

Cardiac muscle is an excitable tissue dependent on K^+ for its normal functioning. The K^+ permeability of the cardiac muscle cell membrane varies directly with plasma $[K^+]$. After excitation, the repolarisation of the muscle is brought about by an increase in K^+ permeability, causing K^+ to move out of the cells. In hypokalaemia, the time for cardiac muscle to repolarise is prolonged. The effect of this on the ECG is shown in Figure 10.1. These characteristic ECG changes appear when plasma K^+ concentration falls to about 3 mM. There is ST segment depression, decreased amplitude (or inversion) of the T wave, a much enlarged U wave and (frequently) arrhythmias. (The arrhythmias of hypokalaemia are more severe in subjects taking digitalis.)

Treatment consists of the oral or intravenous administration of a potassium salt. This must be done with great care, however, since hyperkalaemia can be readily produced. Continual monitoring of the ECG is the best way of monitoring the effect of the K^+ administration. It is difficult to predict the extent of a K^+ deficit, since the plasma $[K^+]$ is a poor guide to K^+ depletion. In fact, because acidosis causes the release of K^+ from cells, it is possible for the plasma $[K^+]$ to be elevated in a patient who is K^+ depleted. Similarly, in alkalosis, the entry of K^+ into cells can depress the plasma K^+ even in subjects with excess total K^+. Thus assessment of the K^+-balance status of a patient cannot readily be made unless any acid-base disturbances are first corrected.

There are a number of ways in which K^+ can be replaced in potassium

Figure 10.1: Changes in the electrocardiogram (ECG) in disorders of potassium homeostasis (lead aVL recording). (a) Hyperkalaemia, with characteristic peaked T wave and widening of QRS complex (plasma $[K^+]$ = 8 mM). (b) Normal ECG (plasma $[K^+]$ = 4 mM). (c) Hypokalaemia, showing characteristic flattened T wave and ST segment depression. The U wave is often prominent and may be mistaken for the T wave (plasma $[K^+]$ = 2 mM).

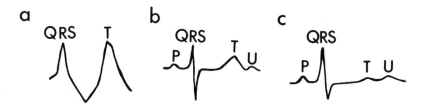

deficit states. Preparations for oral or intravenous administration include KCl, $KHCO_3$ and K_2HPO_4. There are advantages in using KCl, because many K^+-depleted patients are also Cl-deficient (e.g. because of diuretics or vomiting), and have metabolic alkalosis. In a minority of patients who are K^+ depleted and also have metabolic acidosis, $KHCO_3$ is the most appropriate K^+ salt to adminster.

Renal Function in Hypokalaemia

At the onset of hypokalaemia (e.g. if the diet is changed to a K^+-deficient one), the kidney does not immediately conserve K^+ effectively and urinary K^+ output remains greater than about 30 mmoles/day for 2-3 weeks. During this period, the kidney becomes progressively more efficient at K^+ conservation and K^+ output falls below 30 mmoles/day. Thus hypokalaemia and a low urinary K^+ output is indicative of long-standing K^+ depletion, caused by extrarenal factors (e.g. gastrointestinal loss). Hypokalaemia with a normal or high K^+ output indicates that the K^+ depletion has occurred recently, or that the kidney is the *cause* of the hypokalaemia.

The polyuria and inability to produce concentrated urine, which are usually present in hypokalaemic subjects, are due to:

(1) diminished medullary concentration gradient;
(2) resistance of the collecting ducts to the effects of ADH;
(3) polydipsia.

Potassium depletion also causes some anatomical alterations within the kidney. In the proximal tubule, the cells may develop numerous vacuoles, and in the interstitial spaces fibrosis may occur. These defects disappear when normokalaemia is restored.

Hyperkalaemia

Excess K^+ is normally removed from the body by renal secretion. Ingestion of excess K^+ causes a small rise in plasma $[K^+]$ ('buffered' by the entry of K^+ into cells), and the increased plasma $[K^+]$ stimulates the release of aldosterone from the adrenal cortex, which promotes K^+ secretion. It is rare for excess input of K^+ to present problems. Normal subjects can tolerate tenfold increases in K^+ intake (such as the transfusion of stored blood which may contain 30 mM K^+). However, patients with impaired kidney function, or infants, may suffer hyperkalaemia which can be fatal.

As mentioned above, acidosis can cause hyperkalaemia even when the body's K^+ stores are normal. Insulin promotes K^+ entry into cells, so insulin deficiency can lead to hyperkalaemia. Another cause of hyperkalaemia is the excessive breakdown of cells, e.g. after severe trauma, or treatment with cytotoxic drugs.

Hyperkalaemia can occur as a result of decreased K^+ excretion; in renal failure, as the number of effective nephrons decreases, K^+ excretion per functioning nephron increases, so that K^+ balance can be maintained. However, when renal failure reaches the stage where a reduction in urine flow occurs, K^+ excretion falls and hyperkalaemia develops. The reduction in the kidneys' ability to excrete K^+ in oliguric renal failure is probably due to decreased fluid (and Na^+) delivery to the distal K^+-secreting site.

The reduced intracellular:extracellular $[K^+]$ ratio which occurs in hyperkalaemia, decreases (i.e. makes less negative) the potential across cell membranes and, in excitable cells (nerve and muscle), if the depolarisation reaches the threshold, the cells are unable to conduct further action potentials and muscle weakness (and in extreme cases, paralysis) ensues. This is a characteristic feature of hyperkalaemia, as are ECG changes (Figure 10.1). The use of K^+-sparing diuretics (see Chapter 14), or the presence of renal failure, may exacerbate hyperkalaemia.

Several methods of treatment are possible. Loop diuretics can be used (Chapter 14) to promote K^+ excretion, or insulin (or glucose, which increases insulin release) can be administered, to promote K^+ entry into cells.

The *effects* of hyperkalaemia on muscle function can be corrected even in the continuing presence of hyperkalaemia, by administering Ca^{++}. This makes a larger depolarisation necessary to reach threshold, so can return cell excitability towards normal. The effects of Ca^{++} are transient, so it can be used as a short-term measure while waiting for insulin, for example, to take effect.

Suggestions for Further Reading

Gabow, P. 'Disorders of potassium metabolism' in R.W. Schrier (ed.), *Renal and Electrolyte Disorders* (Little, Brown and Co., Boston, 1976), pp. 143-65

Gennari, F.J. and J.J. Cohen. 'Role of the kidney in potassium homeostasis: lessons from acid-base disturbances', *Kidney Int.*, *8* (1975), pp. 1-5

Lifschitz, M.D., R.W. Schrier and I.S. Edelman. 'Effect of actinomycin D on aldosterone-mediated changes in electrolyte excretion', *Am. J. Physiol.*, *224* (1973), pp. 376-80

Young, D.B. and R.E. McCaa. 'Role of the renin-angiotensin system in potassium control', *Am. J. Physiol.*, *238* (1980), pp. R359-63

11 RENAL REGULATION OF BODY CALCIUM AND PHOSPHATE

Introduction

Calcium is the most abundant cation in the body, there being about 25 moles (1 kg) in an average 70 kg man. Almost all of this calcium is within bone, which consists essentially of complex salts of calcium and phosphate. However, both calcium and phosphorus (as phosphate) have important extra-skeletal functions.

Calcium

Precise control of the extracellular fluid (including plasma) calcium concentration is necessary because of the effects of calcium on excitable tissues (nerve and muscle). The excitability of nerve and muscle cell membranes depends on the difference between the resting membrane potential and the threshold potential. The threshold potential varies inversely with the plasma Ca^{++} concentration.

In fact, calcium is present in two forms in the plasma:

(1) Ionised calcium, Ca^{++}, normally about 1.25 mmol/ℓ (5 mg/ 100 mℓ).
(2) Bound calcium. This is mainly bound to protein (especially albumin), but some is complexed with organic acids. The bound calcium concentration is also about 1.25 mmol/ℓ.

Physiologically, the ionised calcium is the more important, but generally, measurements of plasma calcium are of *total* calcium, for which the normal value is about 2.50 mmol/ℓ. It should be noted though that this value is *not* for the ECF as a whole, since the interstitial fluid will have very little bound calcium (there being only a small amount of protein in the interstitial fluid), so interstitial fluid *total* calcium is close to 1.25 mmol/ℓ.

Maintenance of Calcium Balance

Figure 11.1 shows the normal dietary intake and faecal and urinary

138

Figure 11.1: Daily calcium intake and output. All figures are grams. Functionally, the calcium in the body can be divided into three pools, labelled a, b, c. (a) The gut. This normally receives 1 g calcium per day in the diet, and about 700 mg of this is absorbed. However, the net reabsorption is only 100 mg, since 600 mg re-enters the gut. Thus the faeces contain 900 mg calcium per day. (b) The 'pool' of exchangeable calcium. About 5 g calcium in the body is 'exchangeable'. This is present on bone surfaces (2 g) and in the body fluids (3 g). Exchanges occur between this compartment and the gut, and also between this compartment and the 'stable calcium'. (c) Stable calcium in bone. There is about 1,000 g of this, but only 0.5 g exchanges daily with the 'exchangeable' calcium pool. Losses of calcium from the exchangeable pool occur normally in the urine. During pregnancy and lactation there are additional requirements for calcium, and net gut absorption increases.

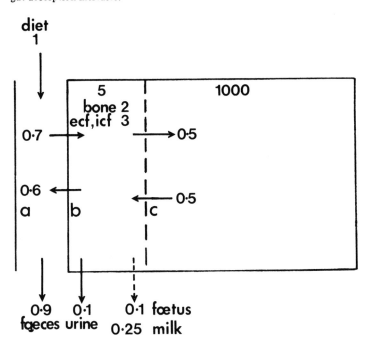

losses of calcium. Normally, the urinary loss per day is equal to the net intestinal absorption.

Calcium Handling by the Kidney

Approximately 50 per cent of the plasma calcium is bound to plasma protein and is therefore not filterable. The remainder (mainly ionised calcium) is filtered, but normally less than 5 per cent of the filtered calcium appears in the final urine. Since the plasma ionised calcium concentration is 1.25 mmol/ℓ, the amount filtered per day is 1.25 x 180 mmol, i.e. 225 mmol. Of this, about 215 mmol is reabsorbed.

Proximal Tubule. Calcium reabsorption in the proximal tubule parallels the reabsorption of sodium and water, and the calcium concentration therefore stays approximately constant along the proximal tubule.

Since Ca^{++} is positively charged, there are, energetically, no problems in the entry of calcium into the cell. But, at the peritubular side, the nature of the transport process is still not clear. A calcium-activated ATPase has been demonstrated in the peritubular cell membrane, but in addition, dependence on the presence of sodium may exist, in which case Ca^{++} counter-transport out of the cell, coupled to passive Na^+ entry, may occur, the energy being derived from active sodium transport which maintains a low intracellular Na^+ concentration.

Loop of Henle. In the ascending limb of the loop of Henle, calcium reabsorption occurs, but it is not clear whether this is independent or secondary to active chloride transport. Furosemide, a diuretic which acts primarily by inhibiting active NaCl transport in the loop of Henle, also inhibits calcium reabsorption.

Distal Tubule and Collecting Duct. Normally, 10-12 per cent of the filtered load of calcium is delivered to the distal tubule (this is the same proportion as for sodium), and about two-thirds of this calcium is reabsorbed. The lumen of the tubule in this part of the nephron is negative (see p. 71), so active calcium absorption is thought to occur, against the electrochemical gradient.

Phosphate

Inorganic phosphate exists in the plasma and interstitial fluid in two forms, 'acid' phosphate $H_2PO_4^-$ and 'alkaline' phosphate $HPO_4^=$. A third form, $PO_4^{\equiv}$ can exist, but does not occur at physiological pH. Generally the term 'phosphate' is used to refer to all of these forms.

Inside the cells, phosphate is present not only as 'acid' and 'alkaline' inorganic phosphate, but also in organic molecules such as ATP, ADP and cyclic AMP. In the extracellular fluid, the proportions of the two forms of inorganic phosphate are determined by the pH. The pK for the interconversion of the forms,

$$H_2PO_4^- \rightleftharpoons H^+ + HPO_4^=$$

is 6.8, i.e. at pH 6.8 $[HPO_4^=] = [H_2PO_4^-]$. However, since the normal plasma pH is 7.4, there will be more $HPO_4^=$ than $H_2PO_4^-$, the ratio being 4:1.

This can be derived from the Henderson-Hasselbalch equation (see Chapter 9) where

$$pH = pK + \log \frac{[base]}{[acid]} \text{, so for phosphate}$$

$$7.4 = 6.8 + \log \frac{[HPO_4^=]}{[H_2PO_4^-]}$$

$$\log \frac{[HPO_4^=]}{[H_2PO_4^-]} = 0.6$$

$$\therefore \frac{[HPO_4^=]}{[H_2PO_4^-]} = \frac{4}{1}$$

Maintenance of Phosphate Balance

Phosphate is filtered at the glomerulus into the nephrons, so that the 4:1 ratio of alkaline to acid phosphate is present in the glomerular filtrate. Conversion of alkaline to acid phosphate occurs in the tubules as a result of H^+ secretion (see Chapter 9).

The phosphate present in the plasma is normally expressed as an amount of elemental phosphorus (P). The normal range is 0.8-1.3 mmol/ℓ. At a concentration of 1.0 mmol/ℓ phosphorus, almost all (95 per cent) of the filtered phosphate is reabsorbed. This reabsorption mainly occurs in the early proximal tubule.

The only hormone which is definitely known to regulate renal tubular phosphate transport physiologically is PTH (parathyroid hormone), although other peptide hormones — notably calcitonin, glucagon and insulin — may also influence renal phosphate transport. Generally, PTH, calcitonin and glucagon increase renal phosphate excretion, whereas insulin reduces phosphate excretion.

Calcium and Phosphate Homeostasis (Refer to Figure 11.1)

Calcium and phosphate can enter the ECF from:

(1) the intestine (via dietary intake);
(2) bone stores;

and can leave the ECF:

(1) via the kidneys (in urine);
(2) into bone.

There is an inverse relationship between plasma calcium and phosphate concentrations, because $[Ca^{++}]$ x [phosphate] is close to the solubility product, so an increase in $[Ca^{++}]$ will cause the precipitation of calcium phosphate (in bone), thus lowering the phosphate concentration. Similarly an increase in phosphate concentration lowers the calcium concentration. But *small* changes in plasma calcium may lead to *parallel* (rather than inverse) changes in plasma phosphate. Nevertheless, the mechanisms whereby calcium and phosphate are regulated are closely interrelated. The two major regulators of calcium and phosphate in the body are parathyroid hormone (PTH) and vitamin D.

Parathyroid hormone is a polypeptide secreted from the parathyroid glands. Secretion is stimulated by a decrease in the plasma ionised calcium concentration, and reduced by an increase in the plasma ionised calcium concentration. Changes in phosphate concentration also change PTH secretion, but this may occur as a result of consequent changes in Ca^{++}. Figure 11.2 shows the main actions of PTH.

Vitamin D is a steroid, cholecalciferol. It is derived from precursors which can be either ingested in the diet or produced by ultraviolet light acting on the skin. The active hormone, 1,25-dihydroxycholecalciferol, is produced by a series of metabolic steps in the liver and kidneys. Essentially its action is to increase the availability of calcium and phosphate by enhancing their intestinal absorption and their release from bone (in the presence of PTH), but it may also reduce the urinary excretion of calcium and phosphate (Figure 11.3). Whereas the single most important action of PTH is on bone, that of vitamin D is on the intestine.

There is a third humoral agent involved in the control of calcium phosphate; this is calcitonin, a peptide hormone which is produced by the parafollicular cells of the thyroid gland. Its effect is to decrease the

Figure 11.2: The actions of parathyroid hormone (PTH).

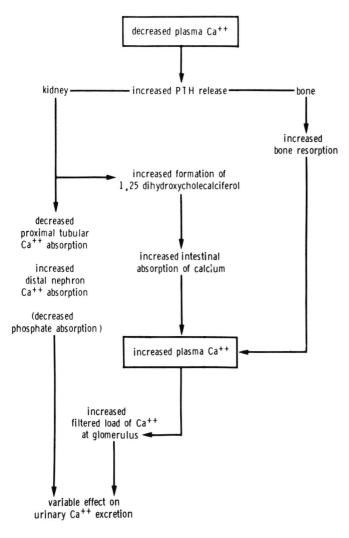

Figure 11.3: The actions of Vitamin D.

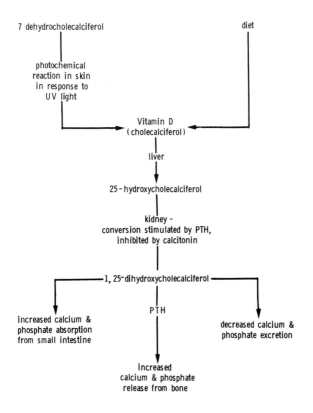

extracellular fluid calcium concentration by reducing the release of calcium from bone.

Disturbances of Calcium and Phosphate Homeostatis

Hypocalcaemia. The characteristic feature of a low plasma [Ca^{++}] is tetany — convulsions, and muscle cramps involving the hands and feet. For nerve and muscle excitability, it is the *ionised* calcium which is important, so it is possible for a severe disturbance to be present even if the *total* plasma calcium is normal. Such disturbances can occur as a result of acidosis or alkalosis. Normally, as we have seen above, the plasma has equal concentrations of bound and ionised calcium. The bound calcium depends on electrostatic charge for its binding (the binding is to the negative charges on the protein molecules). Acidosis causes increased H^+ binding to the negative binding sites on the proteins, so less Ca^{++} can be bound and free $[Ca^{++}]$ rises. Alkalosis has the opposite effect, leading to a fall in free $[Ca^{++}]$, so the symptoms of hypocalcaemia appear even though the *total* plasma calcium is normal.

Conversely, it is possible for the total plasma calcium to be low, without any symptoms of hypocalcaemia. This occurs in hypoalbuminaemia, where the regulatory mechanisms (PTH, vitamin D, calcitonin) keep the plasma ionised calcium concentration normal, but, because the amount of albumin is reduced, the amount of calcium bound to the albumin is also reduced.

Hypocalcaemia is a common finding in patients with renal failure. It is apparently due mainly to hyperphosphataemia and bone resistance to PTH. The amount of phosphate excreted is the difference between the amount filtered and the amount reabsorbed. In renal failure the amount reabsorbed is often normal, but GFR is reduced and hence phosphate excretion is diminished. The plasma phosphate concentration rises, and since $[Ca^{++}]$ x [phosphate] = constant in this situation (see above) there is hypocalcaemia. (This occurs as a result of the deposition of calcium phosphate salts in bone.) PTH release increases, but in severe renal failure may be unable to increase phosphate excretion sufficiently to lower the plasma phosphate concentration (this is true for GFR values of less than 30 ml/min) and deposition of calcium and phosphate may then occur in sites other than the skeleton (e.g. muscle, blood vessels, the heart). This is termed metastatic calcification.

Hypercalcaemia. This can occur as a result of sudden acidosis (see above), releasing 'bound' calcium to become ionised Ca^{++}, so that symptoms of hypercalcaemia occur even though total plasma calcium is normal. True hypercalcaemia (increases in both ionised and bound calcium) can occur as a result of increased intestinal absorption (due to excess vitamin D), or increased release of calcium from bone due to bone disease, or excess PTH, or substances with actions like PTH released from tumours (such as carcinoma of the bronchus).

A major symptom of hypercalcaemia is renal calculi, but in addition there may be disturbances of behaviour (due to effects on higher cerebral function), disturbed intestinal motility and renal damage (due to a toxic effect of calcium on the renal tubules). There may be calcification in extra-skeletal sites.

Suggestions for Further Reading

Agus, Z.S., L.B. Gardener, L.H. Beck and M. Goldberg. 'Effects of parathyroid
hormone on renal tubular reabsorption of calcium, sodium and phosphate',
Am. J. Physiol., *224* (1973), pp. 1143-8
Avioli, L.V. and J.G. Haddad. 'Vitamin D: current concepts', *Metabolism*, *22*
(1973), pp. 507-31
Massry, S.G. and H. Fleisch (eds). *Renal Handling of Phosphate* (Plenum Medical
Book Co., New York and London, 1980)
Mühlbauer, R.C., J.-P. Bonjour and H. Fleisch. 'Chronic thyroparathyroidectomy
and tubular handling of phosphate', *Pflügers Arch.*, *388* (1980), pp. 185-9
Poujeol, P., R.L. Jamison and C. de Rouffignac. 'Phosphate reabsorption in
juxtamedullary nephron terminal segments', *Pflügers Arch.*, *387* (1980), pp.
27-31

12 A SUMMARY OF THE PRINCIPAL REABSORPTIVE AND SECRETORY PROCESSES IN THE NEPHRON SEGMENTS

Introduction

In the foregoing chapters, the major ways in which solutes and water are reabsorbed and secreted along the nephron have been reviewed. In this chapter, the data are summarised. However, although an attempt has been made to relate the amounts of sodium and water absorbed to the GFR in *man*, the data for the segmental absorptions are determined by micropuncture techniques which cannot be used in man and the figures presented must therefore be regarded as approximations.

Sodium

Table 12.1 shows the extent of sodium reabsorption along the nephron.

Changes in sodium reabsorption in the collecting duct provide the fine control of sodium excretion in normal circumstances. It is likely that glomerulotubular balance keeps the delivery of sodium to the collecting ducts approximately constant.

Water

The pattern of water reabsorption along the nephron has some important differences from that of sodium. In the presence of normal amounts of plasma ADH (such that urine volume is about 1.5 ℓ/day), it can be seen (Table 12.2) that there is water reabsorption along with Na^+ in the proximal tubule, but that there is less water reabsorption (as a percentage of the amount filtered) than Na^+ absorption in the loop of Henle. This is because NaCl extrusion from the ascending limb of Henle is not accompanied by H_2O reabsorption (the ascending limb is impermeable to water). The water reabsorption occurring in the loop of Henle is mainly from the descending limb, into the hypertonic medullary interstitium.

The water permeability of the distal tubule is low, and is not affected

147

Table 12.1: Segmental sodium reabsorption.

Segment	Approx. % Glomerular Filtrate Reabsorbed	Amount Na Reabsorbed/Day (mmoles)
proximal tubule	70	17,800
loop of Henle	20	5,200
'distal tubule' and collecting ducts	9	2,200
Total	99	25,200

Table 12.2: Segmental water reabsorption.

Segment	% Glomerular Filtrate Reabsorption	
	Normal ADH Present	ADH Absent
proximal tubule	70	70
loop of Henle	5	4
'distal tubule' and collecting ducts	24	13
Total	99	87
Volume excreted	1.5 ℓ/day	23 ℓ/day

by changes in plasma ADH level. Nevertheless, water reabsorption occurs here to a greater extent than Na^+ reabsorption, because the fluid entering the distal tubule is hypotonic to plasma (as a result of the NaCl extrusion in the ascending limb of Henle). So there is an osmotic gradient for distal tubular water reabsorption, which is therefore largely independent of local sodium reabsorption.

In the collecting ducts, water reabsorption is dependent on ADH; most of the water (66 per cent) delivered to the collecting ducts is reabsorbed in the *cortical* part of the duct, and the tubular fluid osmolality here increases from 100 mosmoles/kg H_2O to almost 300 mosmoles/kg H_2O. In the medullary collecting ducts, water reabsorption continues leading to the excretion of hypertonic urine.

In the absence of ADH, water reabsorption is modified, not only in the collecting ducts, but also (to a lesser extent) in the loop of Henle. The impermeability of the collecting ducts to water (including the cortical collecting ducts), causes the excretion of a large volume (23 ℓ/day) of hypotonic urine. Since Na^+ reabsorption occurs in the collecting ducts, urine osmolality can be as low as 60 mosmoles/kg H_2O. An additional consequence of the absence of ADH is that the medullary tissue osmolality is reduced (due mainly to the washout of urea by the vasa recta and the fact that the rate of urea entry to the medulla from the collecting ducts is reduced). This reduced medullary interstitial osmolality decreases the gradient for water reabsorption from the descending limb of the loop of Henle, so that reabsorption in this segment is somewhat reduced.

Potassium

About 80 per cent of the filtered potassium is reabsorbed in the proximal tubule, and reabsorption continues in the loop of Henle. Most of the potassium which appears in the urine arrives there by secretion from the distal tubule. The collecting ducts are, however, also capable of transporting K^+, either reabsorbing it or secreting it depending upon the requirements of the body.

Hydrogen Ions and HCO_3^-

H^+ secretion occurs in the proximal tubule (active), the distal tubule (active) and the collecting tubule ducts (active). In the proximal tubule, H^+ secretion is responsible for HCO_3^- reabsorption, and there is only a 'small' reduction in tubular fluid pH (from 7.4 down to approximately 7.0). About 10 per cent of the filtered HCO_3^- is still unreabsorbed by the beginning of the distal tubule. H^+ secretion leads to the reabsorption of almost all of this, although there is little carbonic anhydrase activity in the lumen of the distal tubule. Alkaline phosphate is also converted to acid phosphate by tubular H^+ secretion (mainly distal) and the tubular fluid pH decreases. The biggest fall in pH occurs in the collecting ducts, and urinary pH can be as low as 4.5. This demands the maintenance of a very steep plasma-to-lumen H^+ gradient by the collecting duct cells (an $[H^+]$ 1,000 times greater in the lumen than in the plasma), and active H^+ secretion is essential for this.

Phosphate

Ninety per cent of filtered phosphate is reabsorbed in the proximal tubule, at least partly by active transport. Parathyroid hormone inhibits phosphate reabsorption.

Calcium

Only 50 per cent of plasma calcium is filterable; the rest is bound to proteins etc. and is unable to cross the glomerular filter. The filtered calcium (Ca^{++}) is reabsorbed throughout the nephron, and this reabsorption appears in some parts of the nephron (proximal tubule, medullary ascending limb of Henle) to be linked to NaCl reabsorption.

Parathyroid hormone (PTH) affects calcium reabsorption. It decreases proximal Ca^{++} reabsorption, but increases reabsorption in the distal nephron, so that overall it increases tubular Ca^{++} reabsorption. This tubular action of PTH is usually obscured by the fact that PTH increases the plasma calcium concentration by increasing bone resorption, so that the increased filtered load of Ca^{++} may increase calcium excretion.

Glucose

At physiological plasma glucose concentrations, all of the filtered glucose is reabsorbed in the proximal tubule. Only if the plasma glucose concentration rises dramatically is there glucose excretion in the urine. Recent evidence indicates that some glucose reabsorption can occur in more distal parts of the nephron.

Urea

Proximal tubular water reabsorption increases the luminal urea concentration, so that urea (which is lipid soluble and can freely cross most cell membranes) is passively reabsorbed. In the cortical collecting ducts, urea is unable to escape from the tubular lumen, and consequently, if water is being absorbed (i.e. ADH present), the luminal urea concentration rises. Then, in the medullary collecting ducts (if ADH is present) urea is reabsorbed down its concentration gradient, to achieve a high concentration in the medullary interstitial fluid. This high interstitial concentration causes urea to enter the descending limb of Henle, so there is some recycling of urea from interstitium to descending limb to collecting duct to interstitium.

13 DISEASE CONDITIONS WHICH ALTER RENAL SODIUM AND WATER REABSORPTION

Introduction

A number of disease states alter the renal handling of ions and water. This chapter covers the renal handling of ions (mainly sodium) and water in the following conditions:

(1) congestive heart failure;
(2) shock;
(3) hypertension;
(4) liver disease;
(5) nephrotic syndrome.

In all except the last of these conditions (and possibly also in some forms of hypertension), altered renal function can be regarded as essentially a *compensatory* response, to maintain effective circulating volume. Before considering these disorders, it is necessary to consider the factors which can alter the balance between the formation and reabsorption of tissue fluid.

Oedema

Oedema is an increase in the interstitial fluid volume, so that swelling of the tissue results. There are many clinical states which lead to oedema, but the immediate cause is always a change in the rate of formation or reabsorption of tissue fluid, such that the rate of formation exceeds the rate of reabsorption. The formation of tissue fluid depends on Starling's forces (Chapter 1), so that

$$\text{Net formation of tissue fluid} \propto \begin{bmatrix} \text{forces favouring} \\ \text{filtration out of} \\ \text{capillary} \end{bmatrix} - \begin{bmatrix} \text{forces opposing} \\ \text{filtration out of} \\ \text{capillary} \end{bmatrix}$$

$$\propto (P_{\text{cap}} + \Pi_{\text{if}}) - (\Pi_{\text{cap}} + P_{\text{if}})$$

(where P_{cap} = capillary hydrostatic pressure; P_{if} = interstitial fluid hydrostatic pressure; Π_{cap} = capillary oncotic pressure; Π_{if} = interstitial fluid oncotic pressure). A change in any of these four forces can lead to oedema.

The capillary hydrostatic pressure (P_{cap}) is markedly influenced by alterations in venous pressure. The arterioles, which have a high resistance to flow, ensure that only a relatively small pressure is transmitted from the arteries to the capillaries, and that changes in arterial pressure have little effect on capillary hydrostatic pressure. However, there are no high-resistance vessels between the capillaries and the venous side of the circulation, and consequently changes in venous pressure can have a considerable effect on the capillary hydrostatic pressure.

Increases in capillary hydrostatic pressure will occur, therefore, in any circumstances which increase the venous pressure, e.g. during volume expansion (when an increased intravascular volume increases venous pressure), or when venous return is inadequate (e.g. prolonged standing causes venous pooling in the legs and leads to oedema of the feet and ankles), or when the venous return is obstructed.

The plasma protein osmotic pressure (oncotic pressure, Π_{cap}) opposes the capillary hydrostatic pressure and is responsible for the reabsorption of tissue fluid into the vascular system at the venous end of the capillaries. Volume expansion (e.g. by renal sodium retention), in addition to increasing the capillary hydrostatic pressure (see above), will also tend to dilute the plasma proteins, thereby reducing the force for tissue fluid reabsorption, and exacerbating the oedema. Π_{cap} can also be reduced by albumin loss in the urine, or as a result of decreased plasma protein synthesis by the liver.

Interstitial fluid oncotic pressure (Π_{if}) depends on the protein content of the interstitial fluid, and the capillaries have a very low permeability to plasma proteins. However, small quantities (mainly albumin) do seep across and, in some circumstances, proteins accumulate in the interstitial fluid, and cause oedema. This occurs in conditions of: (a) increased capillary permeability and (b) obstructed lymphatic drainage – the plasma proteins which leak out of the capillaries normally enter the lymphatic system, and are eventually returned to the vascular system via the thoracic duct. Blockage of the lymphatics – e.g. by a tumour, or by parasites (as in elephantiasis) – increases the interstitial oncotic pressure and so causes oedema.

The interstitial fluid hydrostatic pressure (or 'tissue turgor pressure') is very difficult to measure accurately, but is close to zero mm Hg.

Congestive Heart Failure

When the cardiovascular system is failing to provide the normal perfusion of the tissues, renal functional adjustments occur which can be regarded as adaptations to increase the effective circulating volume. Such adjustments occur in congestive heart failure. In this condition, the reduction in cardiac output reduces renal perfusion, and, to the kidney, the effect is *as if* there is hypovolaemia. Here we see the reason for using the term 'effective circulating volume' rather than just 'circulating volume' or 'vascular volume'. In chronic congestive heart failure the vascular volume is normal (or may be elevated) but the effective circulating volume is reduced.

The diminished effective circulating volume has the same effect at the kidney as true hypovolaemia — i.e. it promotes the renal retention of NaCl and water (for mechanism, see p. 104). The extent of this retention will depend on the severity of the heart failure, but if the failure is marked the blood volume expands so much that the limit of venous distensibility is reached and venous pressure then increases. At the same time, the retention of NaCl and water dilutes the plasma proteins and hence reduces the plasma protein osmotic pressure. These two factors (increased venous pressure leading to increased capillary pressure, and decreased plasma protein osmotic pressure) give rise to oedema (see p. 104 and 152 for mechanisms).

However, the oedema is essentially a side effect of a *compensatory renal response*, which increases effective circulating volume. The way in which the increased effective circulating volume is brought about is shown in Figure 13.1 (Starling curves).

It can be seen from the figure that expansion of the vascular volume restores tissue perfusion, by increasing the left-ventricular end-diastolic pressure. However, this may lead to a 'side effect' which outweighs the advantage of the restored tissue perfusion — this side effect is pulmonary oedema. If the left-ventricular end-diastolic pressure rises dramatically, there is a transmission of this increased pressure back into the lungs — i.e. left atrial pressure is increased, as is pulmonary venous pressure, and the pulmonary capillary pressure, leading to pulmonary oedema. In the lungs, tissue fluid formation should not occur (otherwise the alveoli fill with fluid and become ineffective), so in health the forces for reabsorption of tissue fluid are greater than those for formation of tissue fluid, throughout the length of the pulmonary capillaries.

From the foregoing it is apparent that oedema of congestive heart failure occurs as a consequence of the renal retention of NaCl and

Figure 13.1: The way in which an increase in effective circulating volume is
brought about by the kidney in congestive heart failure. An important
determinant of cardiac output is the filling pressure (LVEDP, left-ventricular
end-diastolic pressure). The normal relationship of LVEDP to stroke volume (SV)
is shown by curve A. Point a on this line represents typical normal figures for
LVEDP and SV, i.e. at the LVEDP of 9 mm Hg, SV is 75 ml. In heart failure,
the effectiveness of the cardiac contraction is reduced, and a new relationship
between LVEDP and SV is established (curve B). If there is no change in the
filling pressure, the stroke volume will be reduced to less than 50 ml (point b).
This reduces cardiac output and decreases the effective circulating volume; the
renal response to this is fluid and water retention, which increases the central
venous pressure, which in turn increases the right ventricular filling pressure so
that more blood is expelled by the right side of the heart, in turn increasing the
LVEDP, and so increasing the stroke volume to the value at point c. (Similar
curves can be drawn relating right-side SV and RVEDP (right-ventricular
end-diastolic pressure), but normal RVEDP is approximately 5 mm Hg less than
LVEDP.)

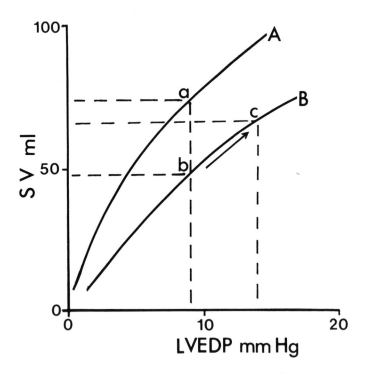

water, to increase the effective circulating volume. This response of the kidney becomes counter-productive if pulmonary oedema occurs. Since it is the heart which is malfunctioning, treatment should logically be directed at the heart — i.e. treatment with digitalis or similar drugs — to restore a more normal cardiac output, although there is no doubt that diuretics do relieve the symptoms of congestive heart failure. However, it should be remembered that systemic oedema is of no danger to the patient, and occurs as part of a compensatory mechanism. Only pulmonary oedema calls for urgent treatment with diuretics to reduce the body fluid volume. Diuretics are definitely advantageous when they reduce pulmonary congestion, but they *also reduce the effective circulating volume.*

The tissue anoxia resulting from circulatory inadequacy in congestive heart failure may cause potassium to leak out of cells and lead to a low total body potassium content before any drug therapy is started. Diuretics may then exacerbate potassium depletion. Furthermore, potassium depletion may occur without being apparent because the plasma potassium concentration can be normal (i.e. the loss is from the cells), and this is important because cellular potassium depletion increases the risk of digitalis-induced arrhythmias.

Hypovolaemia and Shock

Decreases in extracellular fluid volume produced by fluid loss lead to a reduction in cardiac output (due to reduced end-diastolic pressure — Figure 13.1) and, consequently, tissue perfusion is also reduced. The distinction between hypovolaemia and shock is essentially one of degree. Thus the donation of 500 mℓ of blood produces hypovolaemia, but the loss of 1 litre of blood (20 per cent of the blood volume), in addition to hypovolaemia, produces mild shock.

Shock is a life-threatening state with a marked reduction of cardiac output and inadequate perfusion of most organs. Hypovolaemia and mild shock cause tiredness, thirst and dizziness. More severe falls in effective circulating volume are accompanied by signs of increased sympathetic activity (tachycardia, pallor, sweating) and impaired function of vital organs (confusion or coma due to cerebral ischaemia, oliguria (low urine flow) or anuria (no urine flow) and acid-base disturbances due to impaired renal function). There are types of shock in which there is not a reduced blood volume, but all types of shock lead to a reduction in effective circulating volume.

The different mechanisms involved can be grouped under the following headings:

(1) Hypovolaemic Shock. In this type of shock, central venous pressure (CVP) decreases, venous return is reduced and hence cardiac output falls. There are three common causes of hyovolaemic shock:

(1) loss of blood – haemorrhage;
(2) loss of plasma – burns;
(3) loss of fluid – persistent vomiting, severe gastroenteritis, excessive sweating.

(2) Septic or Endotoxic Shock. This is caused by the release of toxins from bacteria (usually from gram-negative bacteria which are normally confined to the gastrointestinal tract). The toxins dilate capillaries and venules, leading to pooling of blood and hence decreased venous return and decreased cardiac output.

(3) Cardiogenic Shock. Sudden reductions in cardic output, e.g. due to myocardial infarction, do not change the intravascular volume, but the venous pressure is increased. This change in venous pressure is in the same direction as occurs in the chronic condition of congestive heart failure. However, the increased central venous pressure (CVP) of cardiogenic shock is a direct consequence of the inability of the heart to pump blood adequately (so right-ventricular end-diastolic pressure is elevated), whereas in congestive heart failure, the increased CVP is more likely to be a consequence of the renal response to inadequate perfusion.

In all three types of shock, both the *effective circulating volume* and the *blood pressure* (b.p.) are reduced. In hypovolaemic shock, the decreased effective circulating volume is due to a decreased ECF volume. In septic (endotoxic) and cardiogenic shock, the decreased effective circulating volume is due to inadequate *circulation*, although the intravascular volume is normal. Exactly what effects the reduction in blood pressure will have on renal function will depend on the magnitude of the reduction. Figure 13.2 shows the autoregulation of renal blood flow (see also p. 85). However, autoregulation means that the kidney is capable of automatic adjustments of its vascular resistance: it does *not* mean that extrinsic influences do not change renal blood flow. When the effective circulating volume is reduced, blood pressure is maintained by increased sympathetic nervous activity (via baroreceptor

Figure 13.2: Autoregulation of renal blood flow. Renal blood flow (RBF) is plotted against mean arterial blood pressure (BP). In the pressure range 90-200 mm Hg, changes in BP have little effect on RBF. This is the 'autoregulatory range'. Below a BP of 80 mm Hg, RBF falls markedly.

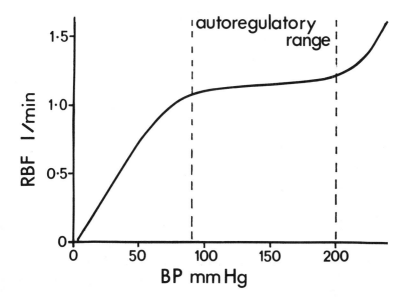

reflexes), which causes vasoconstriction in most parts of the body (except the brain), including the kidney. Thus the sympathetic efferent nerves to the renal arterioles (primarily to afferent arterioles) can over-ride the autoregulatory mechanism and lower the renal blood flow. Nevertheless, the renal blood flow remains adequate (since efferent arteriolar vasoconstriction occurs to maintain filtration pressure) for glomerular filtration, unless the mean b.p. falls below about 80 mm Hg.

Below a mean b.p. of 80 mm Hg, the renal blood flow falls drastically, renal function is impaired, and unless there is prompt restoration of the effective circulating volume, there is the danger of acute renal failure. Let us consider in detail the renal effects of shock, using hypovolaemic shock caused by haemorrhage as an example.

Haemorrhage

Rapid loss of 20 per cent of circulating blood volume produces compensated mild shock. If 30 per cent of the blood volume is lost, there is moderately severe shock (systolic b.p. below 90, heart rate over 90 beats/min), 40 per cent loss causes severe shock, fatal if untreated,

Figure 13.3: The effects of losses of 10, 20, 40 and 50 per cent of the circulating blood volume, on *systolic* blood pressure (BP). Losses of up to 20 per cent of the circulating blood volume have little effect on the blood pressure, although increased sympathetic nervous activity is necessary in order to maintain BP. A loss of 40 per cent of the circulating blood volume lowers blood pressure dramatically, and although increased sympathetic activity can reduce the fall in BP, the degree of vasoconstriction necessary has serious consequences which may lead to death (see text). Larger haemorrhages (50 per cent of circulating blood volume) are more rapidly fatal.

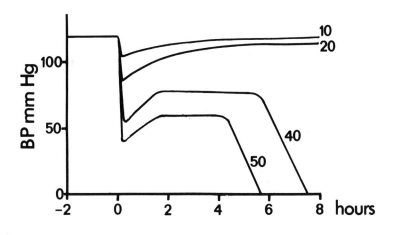

and a loss of over 50 per cent is rapidly fatal (Figure 13.3).

Initially, we will consider the 'compensatory phase' (i.e. where the loss is of less than 20 per cent of the circulating blood volume and the systolic blood pressure remains above 90 mm Hg). In such cases, there is increased sympathetic nervous activity, leading to tachycardia, increased myocardial contractility and peripheral vasoconstriction. These changes serve to maintain blood pressure, since

blood pressure = cardiac output x peripheral resistance

and

cardiac output = heart rate x stroke volume

(Stroke volume is determined by end-diastolic volume and contractility, so increasing myocardial contractility will increase stroke volume even if end-diastolic volume is constant.)

These actions of the sympathetic nervous system, serving to maintain blood pressure, are beneficial in the short term, but can have deleterious effects if prolonged. This is because excessive tachycardia shortens diastolic filling time and impairs coronary blood flow (coronary blood flow is greater during diastole), and prolonged vasoconstriction has the following adverse consequences:

(1) Increased aggregation of blood cells, and consequent increased viscosity and microembolisation.

(2) Hypoxia in the gastrointestinal tract leading to (a) increased fragility of lysosomes (and an increased concentration of lysosomal enzymes in the plasma), and (b) the production of a 'myocardial depressant factor' and a factor depressing the activity of the reticuloendothelial system, so that, within two hours of haemorrhage, the body's ability to destroy bacteria or to break down endotoxins is considerably reduced.

(3) Hypoxia in the liver, leading to failure of glycogenesis and failure to convert protein metabolites to urea. Hypoglycaemia, increased blood lactate levels, and acidosis occur.

(4) Hypoxia in muscle, leading to lactic acidaemia, and increased plasma potassium concentration, which has an adverse effect on cardiac performance.

(5) Modified renal function (see below).

Effect of Haemorrhage on Body Fluid Volume and Composition, and Renal Function

The problems associated with haemorrhage can be divided into two groups:

(1) those due to volume depletion leading to inadequate tissue perfusion;
(2) those due to the electrolyte and acid-base disorders which can accompany volume depletion.

In haemorrhage, the fluid (blood) which is lost is isotonic and thus there is no direct effect on the osmoreceptors. However, haemorrhage increases ADH release via the volume receptors so that water is retained (i.e. osmoregulation becomes subordinated to volume regulation — see Chapter 8).

The main change in renal function after haemorrhage is increased sodium reabsorption. Indeed, increased sodium reabsorption (and hence decreased sodium excretion) is such a characteristic feature of hypovolaemia that it can be used diagnostically. The mechanisms responsible for this decreased sodium excretion have been considered in Chapter 8, but will be briefly reiterated here. Haemorrhage reduces effective circulating volume which then reduces renal perfusion pressure. However, renal sodium conservation occurs before decreases in GFR can be observed, indicating changes in tubular reabsorption. GFR can be maintained in spite of some degree of afferent arteriolar constriction, if the efferent arterioles are also constricted (i.e. there is increased filtration fraction). The peritubular capillary hydrostatic pressure, however, will be reduced, favouring increased sodium reabsorption. In addition, the decreased renal perfusion pressure decreases afferent arteriolar wall tension, and so stimulates the release of renin and the production of angiotensin II which increases adrenal aldosterone release to promote sodium retention. The intrarenal actions of angiotensin II may also favour sodium reabsorption (Chapter 8).

The increased ADH release brought about by the 'volume' receptors in the atria, and by the baroreceptors in the arteries, leads to water retention, so that plasma osmolality decreases (Chapter 8); since the main solute in the plasma is Na^+, this decreased osmolality represents a decreased $[Na^+]$, which therefore acts as a direct stimulus in the adrenal cortex to increase aldosterone release. Extrarenal receptors also modify renal function — decreases in systemic blood pressure reflexly (via the baroreceptors) increase renal sympathetic nerve activity, and this is an additional stimulus to renin release.

In concert, the above mechanisms can reduce the urinary sodium concentration to less than 1 mmol/ℓ. Such effective sodium reabsorption can lead to disturbances of acid-base balance because the reabsorption and excretion of other ions are influenced by sodium reabsorption. The sodium concentration in the glomerular filtrate is 140 mM, whereas the filtrate Cl^- concentration is only about 110 mM. Thus from each litre of glomerular filtrate, only 110 mmoles of Na^+ can be reabsorbed with Cl^- following to maintain electroneutrality. Any additional sodium reabsorption must involve other ways of maintaining electroneutrality, i.e. H^+ and K^+ secretion. Thus

$$Na^+ \text{ reabsorption} \equiv Cl^- \text{ reabsorption} + H^+ \text{ secretion} + K^+ \text{ secretion}$$

So, when sodium is being maximally conserved, K^+ and H^+ are lost from the body, tending to cause *metabolic alkalosis*. However, the acid-base status of subjects with hypovolaemic shock is unpredictable, since inadequate renal perfusion can cause acidosis (see below).

Additional Problems of Severe Haemorrhage (Hypovolaemic Shock). As the degree of hypovolaemia increases, there occurs a stage at which tissue perfusion becomes inadequate. When the perfusion of the kidneys is not sufficient for the maintenance of normal urine flow, H^+ secretion can no longer occur at an adequate rate and *metabolic acidosis* can occur. This is exacerbated by inadequate blood flow to other tissues (e.g. muscle), so that tissue respiration becomes partially anaerobic and lactic acidosis occurs. Restoration of perfusion will correct such acidosis, but HCO_3^- should be administered if arterial pH is below 7.2.

Measures to Prevent Irreversible Renal Damage. In severe volume depletion the stimulus for renal vasoconstriction is so intense that the renal blood flow may not be restored by measures (e.g. blood transfusion) to restore the circulatory volume. Mannitol (an osmotic diuretic – see Chapter 14) may improve renal function, but permanent renal failure can occur due to anoxia and necrosis.

Hypertension

The kidneys contribute to the regulation of blood pressure by regulating the extracellular fluid volume and by releasing vasoactive substances (hormones) into the blood.

In Chapter 8, the renal regulation of ECF volume was discussed. The blood volume is determined by the ECF volume and, since blood volume influences cardiac output, which in turn influences blood pressure, it is clear that ECF volume is a potential determinant of blood pressure. However, changes in blood volume and the consequent changes in blood pressure are normally accompanied by compensatory changes in renal sodium and water excretion, so the persistence of a high blood pressure (i.e. hypertension) may indicate the presence of a disturbance in the kidneys' response to the increased pressure.

In some types of hypertension (secondary hypertension) the causes of this abnormal responsiveness of the kidney are known. These include renal artery stenosis (renovascular hypertension), intrinsic renal disease (renal hypertension), primary hyperaldosteronism (leading to renal sodium retention), or excessive renin production (e.g. in some renal tumours).

Secondary Hypertension

(1) Renovascular Hypertension. This is caused by the renal response to reduced renal perfusion (e.g. due to the stenosis of the renal artery or of one of the interlobar arteries). Reduced perfusion of the afferent arterioles stimulates renin release from the juxtaglomerular apparatus, increasing the production of angiotensin II and thereby causing increased blood pressure both directly (via the vasoconstrictor action of angiotensin II) and indirectly (via salt and water retention brought about by angiotensin and aldosterone).

(2) Renal Hypertension. Impaired renal excretion leads to extracellular volume expansion, which can lead to hypertension. In addition, the kidney cortex and medulla synthesise vasodepressor prostaglandins, and although these are thought to have predominately intrarenal functions, they may also have a systemic role in maintaining normotension, so that inadequate renal prostaglandin synthesis could lead to hypertension.

(3) Primary Hyperaldosteronism. This is a rare condition, accounting for less than 1 per cent of hypertension cases. Excessive aldosterone release by the adrenal cortex (usually as a result of an adrenal cortical adenoma) promotes distal nephron sodium reabsorption and potassium secretion. There is normally little or no volume expansion because of 'escape' from the sodium retaining actions of aldosterone (see p. 100). However, there is continued potassium loss, and most patients (90 per cent) with primary hyperaldosteronism have hypokalaemia (with plasma $[K^+]$ less than 3.5 mM). Metabolic alkalosis ($[HCO_3^-]$ greater than 30 mM) may also be present, since H^+ as well as K^+ is lost from the distal tubules. It is not entirely clear why the condition produces hypertension; the degree of volume expansion is seldom large enough to account for the elevated blood pressure. The diagnosis of primary hyperaldosteronism is based on the observations of hypokalaemia, a high rate of aldosterone excretion and low plasma renin activity.

Essential (Primary) Hypertension

In most hypertensive patients there is no obvious cause of hypertension, and this condition is termed essential hypertension. Renal function is usually disturbed (i.e. the kidney is not responding to the hypertension with increased salt and water excretion), but it remains unclear whether the condition is *caused by* abnormal renal function, or whether it *causes* abnormal renal function. Figure 13.4 is a scheme

Figure 13.4: Renal involvement in the regulation of blood pressure. LVEDP = left-ventricular end-diastolic pressure. Alterations of blood pressure lead to changes in the release of renin, angiotensin, aldosterone, prostaglandins and kinins. Starling forces affecting tubular absorption are also changed. The modifications to renal function, to regulate the effective circulating volume, may then alter stroke volume, heart rate and peripheral resistance, which determine the blood pressure. Directional changes (i.e. increases or decreases) are not shown on the diagram, but will be clear from the text and from Chapter 8.

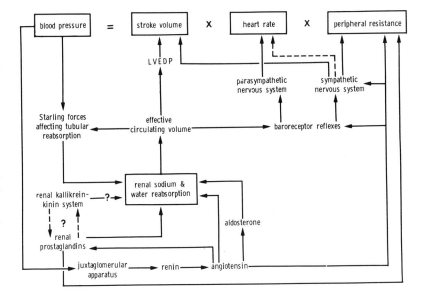

showing the interrelationship of renal function and blood pressure.

About 90 per cent of all hypertensive subjects have 'benign essential hypertension', so called because the condition worsens only gradually. Pathological changes in the kidney in this condition include hypertrophy of the tunica media of the renal afferent arterioles, with consequent narrowing of the vascular lumen (arteriolar nephrosclerosis). Larger vessels (arteries) may also be affected (arteriosclerosis).

In some patients, the hypertension becomes rapidly progressive (malignant hypertension), characterised by extremely high blood pressures (exceeding 230/130 mm Hg), with spontaneous haemorrhages and impairment of the renal blood flow. There is fibrinoid necrosis of the arteriolar walls of many organs, including the kidneys.

Malignant hypertension is almost invariably associated with very high levels of plasma renin, but it is not clear at present whether this is a cause or simply a result of the hypertension and impaired renal blood flow. In benign essential hypertension (even in subjects who subsequently develop malignant hypertension), there are no consistent changes in plasma renin activity.

In summary, if systemic arterial pressure is high, but natriuresis and diuresis are not occurring, then the normal relationship between afferent arteriolar pressure and diuresis does not apply. Has the altered pressure-natriuresis relationship caused hypertension, or occurred as a consequence of it? This question cannot be answered at present, and for a detailed consideration of the evidence, more specialised literature should be consulted (e.g. Birkenhager and Schalekamp, 1976).

Liver Disease

It is a common clinical observation that patients exhibiting symptoms of liver disease − such as jaundice, ascites or portal venous hypertension − frequently develop oliguria (reduced urine flow), sodium retention, or other symptoms of disordered renal function.

How does liver disease lead to disorders of kidney function? The accumulation of oedema fluid in the peritoneal cavity is termed *ascites*, and frequently occurs when there is more general oedema (e.g. in heart failure), but it is a particular feature of abnormal liver function, as its usual cause is an increased hydrostatic pressure in the hepatic portal vein. The hydrostatic pressure in this vessel increases when there is an obstruction within the liver, and the raised pressure forces fluid out of the intestinal capillaries into the peritoneal cavity. It is also possible for ascites fluid to form by transudation from the sinusoids within the liver if the hepatic vein is obstructed.

A potentiating factor in the development of ascites in liver disease is decreased albumin synthesis (the liver is the source of plasma albumin), so that the plasma protein osmotic pressure decreases. The loss of part of the circulating volume by transudation from the capillaries into the peritoneal cavity decreases the effective circulating volume and leads to a renal compensatory response − increased NaCl and water reabsoprtion. A proportion of the fluid thus retained itself becomes ascites.

As the ascites develops, the intra-abdominal pressure rises, and raises the venous pressure in the veins which pass through the abdomen. Thus, the venous drainage of the lower limbs becomes impaired and oedema of the lower extremities develops. Patients with ascites may also have arteriovenous fistulas within the liver, so that the effective circulating

Figure 13.5: The development of ascites in liver disease.

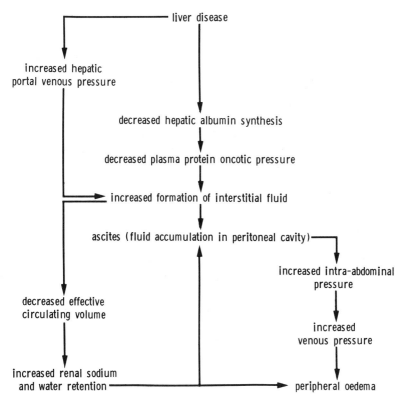

volume is further reduced (since blood passing directly from arteries to veins is not effectively perfusing the tissues).

The development of ascites in liver disease is shown in Figure 13.5. The cautionary remarks concerning the use of diuretics in congestive heart failure also apply to their use in hepatic disease. There is no logical reason why ascites fluid needs to be *rapidly* removed. Its removal should be a gradual process, since part of the accumulation was in response to renal compensatory mechanisms maintaining effective circulating volume. The rapid removal of ascites fluid by a powerful diuretic could catastrophically decrease the effective circulating volume and in addition produce potassium loss. Electrolyte disturbances in the presence of liver disease can be serious and may lead to coma and death (hepatic coma), commonly due to excessively high levels of ammonia in the blood. The sequence of events is as follows: potassium loss from the body leads to hypokalaemia, and the low extracellular fluid $[K^+]$ causes K^+ to leave the cells and Na^+ and H^+ to move in. When this occurs in the renal tubule cells, the lowered cellular pH stimulates NH_3 production from glutamine. Although much of the ammonia so formed enters the renal tubules and is excreted, some enters the blood and, if the liver is healthy, is converted to urea by the liver. In the presence of a diseased liver, the ammonia produced by the kidneys increases the blood ammonia concentration.

Another way in which liver disease (e.g. cirrhosis) complicates renal function is due to the fact that the liver plays a considerable part in the inactivation of circulating ADH and aldosterone, and this inactivation is less effective in cirrhosis.

Nephrotic Syndrome

In this syndrome, the glomerular filtration barrier becomes permeable to plasma proteins, and consequently there is proteinuria, with a progressive reduction in the plasma protein osmotic pressure (Π_{cap}). Albumin is the smallest plasma protein and therefore is filtered most readily in the nephrotic syndrome, and it is also the protein which

Figure 13.6: Oedema in the nephrotic syndrome.

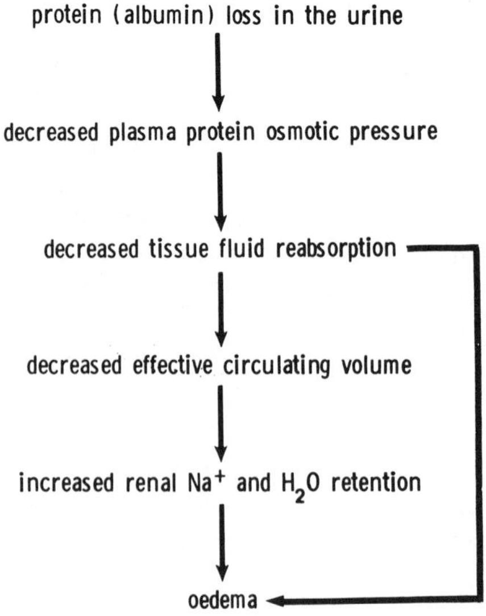

contributes most to the plasma protein osmotic pressure. Thus it is the fall in albumin concentration which is the main cause of the decreased plasma protein osmotic pressure. This in turn alters the 'Starling forces' across the capillaries and causes oedema (Figure 13.6). The reduced effective circulating volume leads to renal sodium and water retention by the same mechanisms as the ones which occur in congestive heart failure.

Suggestions for Further Reading

Birkenhager, W.H. and M.A.D.H. Schalekamp. *Control Mechanisms in Essential Hypertension* (Elsevier, Amsterdam, 1976)

Humes, H.D., M.N. Gottlieb and B.M. Brenner. 'The kidney in congestive heart failure' in B.M. Brenner and J.H. Stein (eds), *Sodium and Water Homeostasis* (Churchill Livingstone, New York, Edinburgh and London, 1978), pp. 51-72

Levy, M. 'The kidney in liver disease' in ibid., pp. 73-116

Mills, I.H. 'Kallikrein, kininogen and kinins in control of blood pressure', *Nephron, 23* (1979), pp. 61-71

Schrier, R.W. 'Renal sodium excretion, edematous disorders, and diuretic use' in R.W. Schrier (ed.), *Renal and Electrolyte Disorders* (Little, Brown and Co., Boston, 1976), pp. 45-77

Wardle, E.N. *Renal Medicine* (MTP, Lancaster, 1979), pp. 57-88

14 THE USE OF DIURETICS

Diuretics are defined as substances which increase the renal excretion of water. There are a number of different chemical types, and there are several possible sites of action for diuretics within the nephron.

Osmotic Diuretics

If the blood glucose concentration rises so that the nephrons are unable to reabsorb all of the filtered glucose, then glucose is excreted in the urine. In addition, the urine flow increases, i.e. diabetes mellitus is usually characterised by the excretion of a large volume of urine, as well as by glucose excretion. Some sodium chloride is also lost and the urinary osmolality is close to plasma osmolality. This is an osmotic diuresis.

Osmotic diuresis can be induced by the intravenous administration of a non-absorbable solute, such as mannitol. The reduction in water (and NaCl) reabsorption which occurs in osmotic diuresis takes place in the proximal tubule and loop of Henle. In the proximal tubule, the normal reabsorptive process does not alter the osmolality of the tubular fluid, which remains at about 290 mosmoles/kg H_2O (isotonic to plasma). Furthermore, the reabsorptive process does not normally change the tubular sodium concentration, since water is reabsorbed at a rate which maintains a constant sodium concentration.

It is thought that the presence of non-reabsorbable solute in the proximal tubule limits water reabsorption, so that sodium reabsorption then lowers the tubular sodium concentration, until the gradient for the passive back-diffusion of sodium into the tubule is such that net sodium reabsorption ceases.

In the renal medulla, osmotic diuretics diminish the corticomedullary osmotic gradient. It has been suggested that this is due to an effect of osmotic diuretics on medullary blood flow (increasing it). However, it is more likely that the effect on blood flow occurs because of the reduced gradient. Thus non-reabsorbable solute in the descending limb of the loop of Henle will limit water absorption, and the chloride concentration in the ascending limb will be reduced, thereby diminishing ascending limb NaCl reabsorption, so that the corticomedullary osmotic gradient diminishes. The diminution of the gradient will reduce the 'short-circuiting' of water between descending and ascending limbs of the vasa recta (p. 74), so that the viscosity of the blood at the tips of the vasa recta loops will decrease and it is likely that this will increase medullary blood flow.

It is not only the renal concentrating ability that is reduced by osmotic diuresis. Diluting ability is also impaired, by the reduced extrusion of NaCl from the ascending limb of the loop of Henle, so that little 'free water' (p. 93) is produced.

Aldosterone Antagonists

Spironolactone competes with aldosterone for receptor sites in the distal tubule (the structures of the two molecules are shown in Figure 14.1). As aldosterone promotes Na^+ absorption and H^+/K^+ secretion, spironolactone causes a natriuresis and reduces urinary H^+ and K^+ excretion. Since its effect is on an ion exchange process, it has little diuretic activity, but its usefulness lies in its ability to reduce the K^+ excretion produced by other diuretics. Thus a combination of, for example, furosemide (see below) and spironolactone minimises the disturbance of K^+ balance which would occur with furosemide alone.

Triamterene and Amiloride

These agents have a similar effect to spironolactone, i.e. they reduce Na^+ absorption and H^+/K^+ secretion in the distal tubule; but they do this by an action which is independent of aldosterone. They have little diuretic action (causing the excretion of only 2-3 per cent of the filtered load), but like spironolactone can be used in conjunction with other diuretics.

Loop Diuretics

Most of the diuretics introduced in the last ten years primarily affect the loop of Henle. Ethacrynic acid, furosemide ('Lasix') and bumetanide are loop diuretics, as are the organomercurials. They act primarily by inhibiting NaCl extrusion from the thick segment of the medullary

Figure 14.1: Chemical structure of a, aldosterone and b, spironolactone.

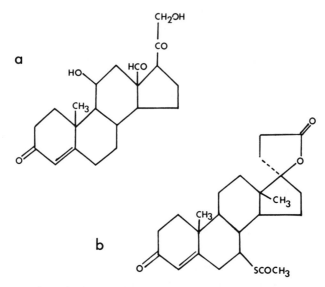

ascending limb, so diminishing the corticomedullary concentration gradient, but there is evidence that they also affect reabsorption of NaCl at other nephron sites. In high doses, furosemide or bumetanide can result in the excretion of over 30 per cent of the filtered load of sodium and water.

Loop diuretics, by increasing the rate of fluid flow in the distal tubule, increase K^+ secretion. The organomercurials have a less dramatic effect on K^+ secretion, but are now (since the introduction of furosemide, bumetanide and ethacrynic acid) seldom used.

Thiazides

The use of thiazide diuretics has diminished since the introduction of loop diuretics, but they are still frequently used in the treatment of hypertension. The thiazides act on the uppermost (i.e. cortical) part of the ascending limb of the loop of Henle and on the early distal tubule. The delivery of sodium to the distal tubular Na^+/K^+ exchange site is increased, so that K^+ secretion is enhanced. Less NaCl is normally absorbed in the cortical ascending limb than in the medullary ascending limb, and consequently the thiazides are less potent than the loop diuretics. They can produce a diuresis of up to 10 per cent of the filtered Na^+ and water.

Carbonic Anhydrase Inhibitors

In the proximal tubule, HCO_3^- is absorbed from the tubule by conversion to CO_2, brought about as a result of H^+ secretion, i.e.

$$HCO_3^- + H^+ \rightleftharpoons H_2CO_3 \rightleftharpoons CO_2 + H_2O$$

The second step in this reaction — the conversion of H_2CO_3 to CO_2 and H_2O — is catalysed by carbonic anhydrase, which is present in the brush border area of the proximal tubule cells. Within the cells, carbonic anhydrase is again necessary to reconvert CO_2 to H^+ (which is secreted) and HCO_3^- (which is reabsorbed). So inhibition of carbonic anhydrase inhibits HCO_3^- absorption from the tubule by blocking the reaction sequence (Figure 14.2) in two places.

The presence in the lumen of non-reabsorbable HCO_3^- reduces Na^+ reabsorption, and $NaHCO_3$ passes into the more distal parts of the nephron. In the distal tubule, K^+ secretion is enhanced, mainly because the delivery of Na^+ to this nephron segment is increased, but also due to the fact that, normally, there is some H^+ secretion (in effect, in competition with K^+ secretion) in exchange for Na^+ reabsorption, and the inhibition of carbonic anhydrase reduces the availability of H^+ for secretion.

Carbonic anhydrase inhibitors are weak diuretics, producing a diuresis which seldom exceeds 5 per cent of the filtered load of Na^+ and water. They are used clinically to correct some acid-base disturbances (alkalosis), rather than for their diuretic action. The inhibitor used clinically is acetazolamide ('Diamox'). Loop diuretics and thiazides also have some carbonic anhydrase inhibitory activity.

The Clinical Use of Diuretics

Some of the dangers of diuretic therapy have been mentioned in Chapter 13, the main point being that oedema is almost invariably a *symptom* of another disorder and not a disease in itself. Furthermore, systemic oedema (as opposed to pulmonary oedema) is not an immediate threat to the life of the patient and there is seldom any justification for the *rapid* removal of oedema fluid. Indeed there are often good

Figure 14.2: Impairment of HCO_3^- reabsorption by carbonic anhydrase inhibitors. The reaction sequence is blocked at the two points shown by xxxx.

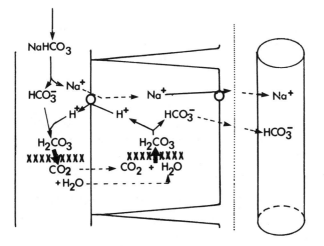

reasons for caution in eliminating oedema rapidly.

In chronic congestive heart failure (Chapter 13), oedema is a consequence of renal fluid retention, and this fluid retention is a compensatory response to increase the effective circulating volume. Diuretic therapy to reduce the oedema will also reduce the effective circulating volume, which may, if the heart failure is severe, be barely adequate. Nevertheless, diuretic therapy, if carefully monitored, is generally beneficial in most patients, since some pulmonary congestion is usually present and diuretic therapy reduces this.

Apart from diminution of the effective circulating volume, other disturbances which can be produced by diuretics are:

(1) Acid-base and Electrolyte Disturbances. Diuretics which cause NaCl excretion (furosemide, ethacrynic acid and thiazides) can produce metabolic alkalosis, because they increase the delivery of NaCl to the distal exchange site where Na is absorbed and K^+ and H^+ are secreted. Thus both alkalosis and hypokalaemia ensue. The alkalosis is exacerbated by the contraction in body fluid volume brought about by the diuretic, since the HCO_3^- content of the body is essentially unchanged, so that the HCO_3^- concentration increases.

Diuretic agents which act at the distal exchange sites (spironolactone and triamterene) reduce H^+ and K^+ secretion, so their use can result in hyperkalaemia and metabolic acidosis.

(2) Azotaemia and Hyperuricaemia. If diuretic administration leads to a reduction in effective circulating volume, then renal perfusion may be reduced, with a consequent fall in urea and creatinine excretion.

Hyperuricaemia can occur because proximal tubular sodium reabsorption determines the extent of uric acid reabsorption. Diuretics with actions distal to the proximal tubule will, by causing volume depletion, actually *enhance* proximal sodium absorption and uric acid reabsorption will also be enhanced.

Suggestions for Further Reading

Burg, M.B. 'Mechanisms of action of diuretic drugs' in B.M. Brenner and F.C. Rector (eds), *The Kidney*, vol. 1 (Saunders, Philadelphia, London, Toronto, 1976), pp. 737-64

Grantham, J.J. and A.M. Chonko. 'The physiological basis and clinical use of diuretics' in B.M. Brenner and J.H. Stein (eds), *Sodium and Water Homeostasis* (Churchill Livingstone, New York, Edinburgh, London, 1978), pp. 178-211

INDEX

174